NA

Le___Roots
Be Your
Medicine

N H Hawes

BOOKS

Hammersmith Health Books
London, UK

First published in 2017 by Hammersmith Health Books – an imprint of
Hammersmith Books Limited
4/4A Bloomsbury Square, London WC1A 2RP, UK
www.hammersmithbooks.co.uk

Note: No book can replace the diagnostic expertise and medical advice of a trusted physician. Please be certain to consult your doctor before making any decisions that affect your health or extreme changes to your diet, particularly if you suffer from any medical condition or have any symptom that may require treatment. Whilst the advice and information in this book are believed to be true and accurate at the date of going to press, neither the author nor the publisher can accept any legal responsibility or liability for any errors or omissions that may have been made.

British Library Cataloguing in Publication Data: A CIP record of this book is available from the British Library.

ISBN (print edition): 978-1-78161-085-5
ISBN (ebook): 978-1-78161-086-2

Commissioning editor: Georgina Bentliff
Cover design by: Julie Bennett, Bespoke Publishing Ltd
Typeset by: Julie Bennett, Bespoke Publishing Ltd
Production: Helen Whitehorn, Path Projects Ltd
Printed and bound by TJ International Ltd

Contents

About Nature Cures

This pocketbook is a guide to natural ways to treat health issues. The information is drawn from my website www.naturecures.co.uk and my comprehensive book *Nature Cures: The A to Z of Ailments and Natural Foods*, available from www.hammersmithbooks. co.uk. For more detail about the nutrients and foods listed in this pocketbook, please do refer to these sources.

In both this book and my comprehensive works the sources of the information I've used are too numerous to list without at least doubling the size; if there is any fact or recommendation that is of concern, please do contact me via www.naturecures.co.uk.

This pocketbook represents a compilation of years of research but is no substitute for visiting a qualified health practitioner so please do consult such, especially your doctor with regard to any prescription medications, before making signficant changes to your diet, lifestyle or health regime.

Other titles in the series include
Nature's Colour Codes
Air-purifying Houseplants
Grow Your Own Health Garden
Recovery from Injury, Surgery and Infection

Introduction

Our ancestors evolved to leave the trees and walk upright approximately 4.4 million years ago. This gave them the evolutionary advantage of access to ground-level foods, such as the nutritious roots of plants, and their teeth evolved in line with this. Chimpanzee diets focused more on fruit whilst gorillas stayed with leaves.

The roots of plants have been consumed by humans as nutritious food and used as natural medicines ever since they evolved. Many have astonishing properties which can heal and treat most human ailments and diseases without the harmful side effects of manufactured drugs, but this has largely been forgotten in recent years due to the availability and ease of use of these modern pharmaceuticals.

Losing this traditional knowledge means we now treat some of nature's most powerful natural antibiotics as weeds and discard them, or spray them with toxic weed killers, forgetting that they provide an abundance of nutrients our bodies need.

Two prime examples are dandelions (*Taraxacum officinale,* page 38) and burdock (*Arctium lappa*, page 26). The roots of both these plants have powerful antibacterial, antifungal and diuretic properties and are protective for the kidneys and liver. It is strange that dandelion and burdock both used to be favourite and very healthy and nutritious beverages in years gone by but have since mysteriously disappeared from our repertoire.

Precisely because the roots of plants grow under the ground they absorb many nutrients from the soil, especially minerals. Many produce tubers which are the storehouses for these nutrients and the sources of buds, from which new plants will grow. However, there is a constant battle with microbes and other organisms in the soil that want to consume these rich stores of nutrients. Plants have evolved in thousands of diverse shapes and structures to find sustenance, reach the sunlight, reproduce and evade the microbes and other organisms that want to feed on them. Their predators have evolved similarly to overcome the obstacles plants place in their way.

Plants have also developed antimicrobial substances to repel or kill off particular invading foragers and parasites. When we consume these substances, they can have a similar effect within and upon the human body. They will destroy the microbes and parasites that also try to feed on us. For instance, garlic and onions produce allicin when damaged, which is a very powerful antioxidant. For the underlying chemical reaction to take place, these roots must be left to stand for 10 minutes after being peeled and chopped, before being cooked or consumed.

Certain roots contain fat-soluble nutrients, such as carotenoids and vitamins A, D, E and K; these nutrients will not be absorbed by humans unless they are consumed at the same time as oily food, such as avocado, butter, oily fish or nut, seed and other plant oils. Vitamins D and E are usually found in foods that already contain oils, such as fish, seeds and nuts. Orange-coloured root vegetables, such as carrots, swede and sweet potatores, are especially rich in the carotenoids that are precursors to vitamin A.

How to prepare roots

Unless the outer skins of roots are completely inedible, as in the case of garlic, onions and tough roots such as swedes, the skins should also be consumed as this is often where many of the nutritional or protective compounds are located. Peeling vegetables such as carrots, parsnips, potatoes and sweet potatoes removes many of these vital nutrients and is unnecessary. The skins should simply be scrubbed well before use.

Most roots need either chopping and cooking or drying and grinding into a powder in order to extract the medicinal properties. Decoctions are the most concentrated and powerful of the following methods, followed by tinctures, then infusions. Unless otherwise stated further on, most of the nutrients and medicinal compounds of the roots mentioned in this pocketbook can be consumed using the methods below.

Baking, steaming and boiling
Raw juicing is a good way to obtain the highest levels of nutrients from vegetables without cooking them and destroying important

enzymes. The juices of vegetables such as carrots and beetroot require little digestion, are rich in alkaline elements and provide plentiful, easily absorbed minerals. The juicing process breaks down tough cell walls but it does remove much-needed fibre too. When consumed as a vegetable, some softer roots can be steamed or boiled to break down their tough cell walls. Baking or steaming them retains more of the vitamin and mineral content, which can be lost in the water when they are boiled. On the other hand, using the water they were boiled in, for gravy and soups etc, is one way of consuming those lost nutrients; however, keeping this liquid for later use will degrade the nutritional content and therefore baking or steaming roots is generally a better choice.

Brine pickling

One of the best ways to store and consume many root vegetables is to immerse them in cold water with salt (brine) and allow them to ferment. Brine pickling, also known as lacto-fermentation, is an easy, traditional and the healthiest method of making pickles without using vinegar. Pickles made using this method are alive and rich in probiotics that are needed for a healthy intestinal environment. It is also a very safe way to preserve any excess produce for up to one year. (For information about how to make your own brine pickles see page 114.)

Decoctions

Decoction involves heating in water to produce a concentrated liquor. Roots and barks that are used medicinally are thicker and less permeable than the above-ground parts of plants and need to be boiled to extract their medicinal constituents. The roots should be scrubbed well, then chopped or broken into small pieces. To avoid losing volatile constituents, use a lid over the simmering pan. After cooling down, strain the solid from the liquid and pour the liquid into an air tight container and store in the refrigerator. Decoctions can be taken hot or cold or added to sauces and soups.

Infusions / macerations

Infusions, or teas, are made by infusing plant material in hot water for a short amount of time. Macerations involve the softening and breaking down of plant cell walls using prolonged exposure to a liquid (water or alcohol – the latter makes an 'alcoholic maceration', see page 11). Use approximately one to two teaspoons of dried root powder per cup of cold filtered water. For **alcoholic macerations** the proportions should be 20 parts of alcohol to one part of the plant.

Water-based infusions

- Bring the water to a boil and pour over the root powder.
- Cover the container and allow to steep for 10-20 minutes.

Consume one tablespoon of the mixture three times a day unless otherwise stated. One teaspoon of honey and the freshly squeezed juice of half a lemon may be added to make the infusion more palatable and provide additional healing properties. Infusions may be gently reheated and consumed as a tea with other medicinal herbs and spices.

Infused oils

Pure vegetable oils such as almond, olive, rapeseed and sunflower are easily found at general grocery stores. They have the property of dissolving the active, fat-soluble principles of medicinal plants. This process is called infusion and can be carried out at room temperature or higher. Infusion is a slower process than alcoholic maceration but has the advantage of resulting in an oil-based solution of medicinal constituents that can easily be used to make creams and ointments. Hot infusion is recommended for the harder parts of the plants, such as roots and stems, while cold infusion is more suitable for flowers and leaves.

Juicing and blending

Raw juicing is a good way to obtain the highest levels of nutrients from root vegetables without cooking them and destroying important enzymes. The juices of root vegetables such as carrots and beetroot require little digestion, are rich in alkaline elements and provide plentiful, easily absorbed minerals. The juicing process breaks down tough cell walls but it does remove the much-needed fibre too. A way to keep this fibre is to use a powerful blender instead and these are now available to purchase.

Ointments

Ointments are prepared like hot infused oils, the difference being that herbs are simmered in waxes or fats containing no water. After separating the simmered herbs by squeezing and cooling, the result is a solid mixture of the wax or fat with the medicinal constituents of the plant. Petroleum jelly, soft paraffin wax and bees wax are some common bases used. Ointments form an oily barrier on the surface of injuries and carry the active principles to the affected area.

Tinctures

Most of the volatile components of medicinal roots are soluble in alcohol, while some cannot be extracted by other methods as they are 'hydrophobic' (non-polar and repel water). By immersing dried or fresh roots in alcohol, the active principles are easily extracted at concentrations that exceed those that can be achieved by other methods. Furthermore, ethanol (the form of alcohol humans can drink) is easily evaporated under 50-60°C leaving behind the required components. Highly concentrated solutions, that will last for one to two years, are a convenient way to store and use medicinal plant constituents. Ideally tinctures should be made using pure ethyl (ethanol) alcohol distilled from cereals. However, since this product is not easily available, good quality vodka with at least 45 per cent alcohol can be used. Tinctures are also known as 'alcoholic macerations.

Method

- Clean and chop up the fresh roots.
- Place them in a clean container (preferably glass).
- Use a vodka that has at least 45 per cent alcohol content (also known as 90 per cent proof).
- Add the alcohol at a two to one ratio (that is, two cups of vodka to one cup of fresh roots).
- If using dried roots, use a five to one ratio instead (that is, five cups of vodka to one cup of dried roots).
- Make sure the roots are entirely submerged in the vodka.
- Let the mixture sit for about two weeks.
- Then strain it and pour it into a dropper bottle with an air-tight lid.
- Tinctures are meant to be used as medicine in very small amounts. Shake well and add a few drops to juices, smoothies, soups, teas, water or directly into the mouth when needed.
- If kept sealed in a cool dry place, tinctures can last for many years before losing their medicinal properties.

Note: Use ethanol only. Never use alcohol that is not meant for human consumption such as isopropyl alcohol, methyl alcohol, methylated spirits or any other kind of unknown spirit to make tinctures.

The A-Z of medicinal roots

Over the centuries of human inhabitation of this planet, the sheer diversity of plants and their powerful properties has caused many to be given multiple names, depending on the location. This has caused much confusion even to the botanists of Kew Gardens, the leading botanical institution in the world. Many were once commonly named as a 'wort', which meant it was a medicinal plant, or named for their abilities or for where they were found and botanists have since been trying to categorise them into families and have renamed them scientifically using Latin. Their scientific botanical names are included here in brackets, as well as the many of the other common names they are known by, but what is listed here is by no means comprehensive.

Ajos sacha (*Mansoa alliacea*)

An alcoholic maceration (tincture) of the stem and roots of the ajos sancha is used for rheumatism due to its powerful anti-inflammatory properties which can help to reduce pain, spasms and swellings. It also has components that lower cholesterol and fight free radicals.

Alisma (*Alisma plantago aquatica, Alismatis rhizoma, Alisma orientale*)

Alisma grows worldwide, mostly in shallow water. Its root has an antibacterial action on *Mycobacterium tuberculosis* and *Staphylococcus*. It is also useful for treating *Streptococcus pneumoniae* which can cause bacteraemia (blood poisoning), ear infections, meningitis (infections of the brain and spinal cord), pneumonia (infection of the lungs) and sinus infections and may lead to serious complications, especially for young infants and the elderly. The alisma root can also lower blood pressure, blood sugar and LDL cholesterol levels. It is used in the treatment of acute diarrhoea, fatty liver, oedema, oliguria and nephritis.

Alisma was once thought of as a cure for rabies but this has never been substantiated.

The whole plant is believed to promote conception.

The root is harvested before the plant comes into flower and is dried for later use. A homeopathic remedy is obtained from the fresh root. It is used cooked and is rich in starch. Caution is advised as the root is acrid (bitter) if it is not dried or well-cooked before use.

Alum root (*Heuchera*, American keno root, cranesbill root, crowfoot, dovefoot, spotted cranes bill, wild geranium)

Alum root is a strong astringent used to stop the bleeding of cuts, superficial abrasions and ulcers on the lips. It is used in dilute form as a mouthwash or gargle and has been effective for mouth and throat ulcers. Internally, it is useful as a tea to help ease malaria symptoms, diarrhoea/loose bowels and for excessive mucus in the urinary tract accompanied by frequent urination. A decoction can be made of grated alum root simmered in a litre of water until the liquid has halved, strain then drink when cooled. **Note**: Alum root can cause gastrointestinal irritation if taken in large amounts.

Angelica (*Angelica archangelica*, dong quai)

Chinese angelica has been used for centuries in the Far East as a tonic, spice and medicine. The health benefits come from the plant's root and studies have shown that it has powerful antibacterial properties against *Bifidobacteria, Candida albicans, Clostridium difficile, Clostridium perfringens, Enterococcus faecalis, Eubacterium limosum, Lactobacilli* and *Peptostreptococcus anaerobius*.

Due to angelica's antihistamine properties it is also used to treat allergies. It is also used as a muscle relaxant and painkiller and is beneficial for sufferers of lung diseases such as asthma and bronchitis. Used in conjunction with other herbs, like Asian ginseng, it produces the ability to decrease chest pain in patients suffering from heart disease. Further health benefits of Chinese angelica are its ability to stabilise female hormones, ease the pain of arthritis and lower blood pressure.

Nutritionally it supports the brain, digestive and respiratory systems, calms the central nervous system and balances and strengthens the female reproductive system. It can be taken using all of the following methods:

- Decoction (a teaspoon or tablespoon of cut root simmered in one cup of hot water)
- Dried root (taken directly by mouth or in an infusion)
- Root tincture (submerged in 90 per cent alcohol for two weeks)
- Tea (root steeped in hot water)
- Whole root or root slices (boiled or soaked in wine).

Note: Avoid angelica if taking any type of medication that thins the blood or any hormone therapies or contraceptives.

Asafoetida (*Ferula assa-foetida*, hing)

Asafoetida is the dried latex (gum oleoresin) exuded from the rhizome or tap root of several species of the ferula plant. It is often used as an alternative to garlic and onion for those who cannot tolerate the taste or digest these root vegetables.

It is highly favoured as a spice amongst the Jain and Brahmin Indians. It is also known to eliminate tapeworms. For this purpose, dissolve a teaspoon of dried and ground asafoetida in a glass of water and drink on an empty stomach once a day for three days.

Astragalus root (*Astragalus propinquis,* huang-qi)
Astragalus has been used in Chinese medicine for centuries and is one of the most powerful immune system builders in the world. It can also prevent and slow down tumour growth and reduce cortisol in the body, which is the chronic stress hormone. It can prevent cardiovascular disease and viruses that affect the immune system and help to reduce the symptoms caused by chemotherapy. It also reduces inflammation and has antimicrobial properties. In addition, it can relieve insulin resistance and treat diabetes type-2 naturally and help to stabilise cholesterol levels. This is mostly due to its high content of flavonoids, polysaccharides and saponins.

Balloon flower root (*Platycodon grandiflorus*, jie geng)
Balloon flowers are an herbaceous perennial from the Far East that can be grown in full sun or partial shade in a temperate climate. Changkil saponins, isolated from the roots of the balloon flower, have been found to increase intracellular levels of the antioxidant

glutathione, significantly reducing oxidative injury to the body's cells and minimising cell death and lipid peroxidation. Glutathione is an amino acid found in every cell of all human tissues, with the highest concentrations found in the liver and eyes. It is the body's most potent and important antioxidant because it is within the cell and protects fatty tissues from the damaging effects of free radicals; this is especially important for the brain.

Glutathione also plays a vital part in the detoxification of harmful substances in the liver, such as drugs, pollutants and other toxins, and can chelate (pull out) heavy metals such as lead, mercury and cadmium and eliminate them from the body. This is particularly beneficial to those who may be prone to developing, or have developed, Alzheimer's disease, dementia, multiple sclerosis or Parkinson's disease and those who smoke tobacco.

As an immune system booster and a detoxifier, glutathione can also help the body repair damage caused by aging, burns, drugs, infection, injury, pollution, poor diet, radiation, stress and trauma. It has the potential to fight almost any disease, particularly those associated with aging, as free radical damage is the cause of many of the common degenerative diseases of old age. It is also believed that glutathione carries nutrients to lymphocytes and phagocytes, which are important immune system cells.

Many medications can reduce the production of glutathione in the body and people who have cancer, HIV/AIDS or other very serious diseases are, almost invariably, deficient in glutathione.

Conditions that may be caused/exacerbated by lack of glutathione

- Addictions
- (ADHD) Attention-deficit hyperactivity disorder
- Allergies
- Arthritis
- Asthma
- Autism
- Hair loss and balding
- Bronchitis
- Cancer
- Cataracts
- Chronic fatigue
- Cirrhosis of the liver
- Diabetes
- Erectile dysfunction
- Fibromyalgia
- HIV (AIDS)
- Insomnia
- Low energy
- Low sex drive
- Lupus
- Macular degeneration
- Male infertility
- Memory loss
- Migraines
- Osteoporosis
- Joint and back pain
- Poor eyesight
- Premenstrual tension
- Psoriasis
- Scleroderma
- Schizophrenia
- Wrinkles.

Beetroot (*Beta vulgaris*, Swiss chard, beets)

Beetroot is high in iron content. Consequently, beetroot juice regenerates and reactivates the red blood cells and helps supply the body with fresh oxygen.

Beetroot contains the component betacyanin, which is responsible for its deep red colour and is the essential ingredient that can assist the body with recovery from many ailments.

Regular consumption reduces the risk of heart disease, regulates blood pressure, helps control cholesterol levels, strengthens the lungs, stops the spread of cancer tumours, prevents diseases of liver, kidney and pancreas and treats ulcers in the stomach. It also strengthens the immune system, improves the vision and is good for treating eye redness. It can eliminate hard stools, positively affects the colon, improves bad breath due to indigestion, helps treat acne, creates healthy skin and reduces menstrual pain. It also reduces pain after intense physical training and is a useful refuelling food for tired muscles. Beetroot also helps prevent spina bifida in babies when consumed during pregnancy being high in vitamin B9 (folate). Beetroot is relatively low in calories, with just 43 per 100 grams, so is a useful and nutritious food for those trying to lose weight.

It should be noted that consumption of beetroot can cause the stools to turn deep red and be mistaken for blood but this is just the excretion of the pigment of the beetroot and is normal and harmless.

Significant nutrients in beetroot

- Betacyanin
- Betaine
- Choline
- Carbohydrates
- Fibre
- Omega-3 fatty acids

- Omega-6 fatty acids
- Phytosterols
- Protein
- Vitamin A
- Vitamin B1 (thiamine)
- Vitamin B2 (riboflavin)
- Vitamin B3 (niacin)
- Vitamin B5 (pantothenic acid)
- Vitamin B6 (pyridoxine)
- Vitamin B9 (folic acid)
- Vitamin C (ascorbic acid)
- Vitamin E
- Vitamin P (citrin bioflavonoid)

Minerals in beetroots

- Calcium
- Copper
- Iodine
- Iron
- Magnesium
- Manganese
- Phosphorus
- Potassium
- Selenium
- Sodium
- Sulphur
- Zinc.

Biscuit root (*Lomatium cous, Lomatium dissectum, Lomatium geyeri, Lomatium macrocarpum*, Indian parsley)

Biscuit root is one of the most powerful antibiotic, antifungal and antiviral herbs there is, especially for infections of the eyes and the respiratory and urinary tracts. A member of the parsley family, it is historically one of the most important medicinal plants of the native American Indians, who used it as an internal remedy for bacterial, fungal and viral infections. Several tribes of Indians ate the shoots and roots and some immersed the fresh root in streams to stun fish for harvesting. However, the most important use was as a medicine.

A decoction of the root was taken internally to treat asthma, bronchitis, colds, coughs, hay fever, influenza, ocular infections, pneumonia, throat infections and tuberculosis.

The decoction was also applied externally for cuts, sores and rashes. The raw root was also chewed to relieve a sore throat and used as a poultice for swellings, sprains and rheumatism. It was also used to cure equine (horse) distemper and as a nail fungicide for humans and animals.

Note: It is best to use biscuit root with a liver/urinary stimulant such as dandelion root to help avoid a rash side effect.

Bitter leaf (*Vernonia amygdalina* ewuro, hausas, ironweed, mujonso, onugbu, shiwaka, yorubas)

Bitter leaf is a member of the daisy family and an African herb of which the bark, leaves, roots and stems are used for culinary and medicinal purposes. The washed roots and stalks of the bitter leaf plant can be boiled and a cup of the liquid drunk first thing in the morning before food to expel worms and parasites.

Bitter leaf contains steroid glycosides known as type

vernonioside B1. These compounds possess potent antibacterial, antiparasitic, anti-tumour and anti-inflammatory properties. It also contains vitamins A, B1, B2, C and E.

Note: Bitter leaf should never be harvested from locations near to mines, power stations or road sides as it absorbs heavy metals from traffic pollution and chemical combustion which can then be ingested and cause many ill health effects.

Black cohosh (*Cimicifuga racemose*)

The native Americans used black cohosh to treat snakebite. They also used the root to help ease complaints associated with the skeletal system and for many gynaecological conditions, including menstrual cramps, labour and delivery. It can balance hormones in menopausal women and studies have shown that it contains substances that bind to oestrogen receptors. When combined with other nervine herbs (those that support the nervous system), it provides excellent soothing properties. A tea from the root can soothe a sore throat. Black cohosh contains nutrients that help to maintain the respiratory system and blood vessels. It has also been shown in lab experiments (in vitro) to inhibit microbial activity and can treat intestinal infections such as *Helicobacter pylori*.

Note: Black cohosh should be taken with caution as it can cause an allergic reaction.

Blood root (*Sanguinaria Canadensis*, bloodwort, noon root, Indian plant, Indian red paint, pauson, red Indian paint, red puccoon, red root, sang-dragon, sang de dragon, sanguinaire, sanguinaire du Canada, snakebite, sweet slumber, tetterwort)

The root of this plant has powerful antibacterial properties. It is used to cause vomiting and to empty the bowels. It is also used to treat achy joints and muscles (rheumatism), croup, fever, hoarseness (laryngitis), Lyme disease, nasal polyps, poor circulation in the surface blood vessels and warts and to reduce tooth pain and sore throat (pharyngitis).

Blue cohosh (*Caulophyllum thalictroides*, squaw root, papoose root, blue ginseng, yellow ginseng)

The roots of blue cohosh nutritionally support the female reproductive system. It was used by native Americans to treat menstrual cramps, to suppress profuse menstruation and to induce contractions in labour.

Note: Blue cohosh should be taken with caution as it can cause an allergic reaction and pregnant women should avoid this herb unless it is being used to induce contractions.

Blue flag (*Iris versicolor*, blue iris, dragon lily, flag lily, fleur-de-lis, harlequin blue flag, iris ivy, liver lily, poison flag, snake lily, water flag, wild iris)

Native Americans used the root of this plant to make poultices to treat cuts and burns and chewed it to protect themselves against rattle snake bites. It is also used as a laxative and to relieve fluid retention and bloating. Other uses are to treat chronic rheumatism, colic, enlargement of the thyroid gland, pelvic inflammatory ailments, skin disorders, swelling (inflammation) and weight gain. Some people also use it for liver disorders and to increase bile production.

The medicinal compounds in blue flag are:

- iridin
- isophthalic acids
- resin
- salicylic acids
- tannins
- triterpenoids and
- olatile oils.

Note: Blue flag can have side effects such as headaches, nausea, vomiting and watery eyes and should never be used by pregnant or breastfeeding women, or children.

Burdock root (*Arctium lappa*, greater burdock, beggar's buttons, thorny burr)

The burdock plant needs moist ground and is able to grow without shade. It is a native of the 'Old World' and grows wild throughout England but rarely in Soctland. Very few, if any, other herbs possess more curative powers than this one. It has an ancient history as a reliable herbal aid for blood disorders, ulcers and tumours. The root nutritionally supports joints and other skeletal tissues and the urinary and respiratory systems. It promotes glandular and hormone balance and removes accumulations and deposits around the joints. It is also helpful for treating cancer, dyspeptic complaints, leprosy, liver and gallbladder problems, neurologic disorders, scrofula, syphilis and throat and chest ailments. It is also used as an appetite stimulant and can control blood sugar and cholesterol levels, blood pressure, heart rate and weight and can help to prevent muscle wasting.

Western and Chinese herbal medicine both use burdock for detoxification as it is an excellent blood purifier, expelling toxic products from the blood via the urine. Its root is commonly used for treating 'toxic overload' that leads to the following infections and skin ailments.

- Abscesses
- Acne
- Bites
- Bruises
- Burns
- Eczema and dermatitis
- Furunculosis (boils)
- Herpes
- Impetigo
- Lupus
- Pityriasis
- Psoriasis
- Rashes
- Ringworm.

Place a tablespoon of chopped burdock root into one pint of boiled cold water. Simmer gently for 20 minutes. Strain, cool, keep in a cold place and drink four times a day. The dose for adults is a wineglassful (56 ml or 2 fl oz) three or four times a day. For children, less according to age.

This tea can also be used as a skin and face wash. Apply the cooled tea to the skin with a clean facecloth and rinse in cool water. The leaves can also be crumpled and the seeds crushed to topically treat bruises, burns, sores, stings and ulcers.

Burdock root is very low in calories - 72 calories per 100 grams – and a good source of non-starch polysaccharides such as inulin, glucoside-lappin and mucilage. While being low in sodium, it contains high amounts of electrolyte potassium and many important vitamins and minerals, including vitamin B2 (riboflavin), vitamin B3 (niacin), vitamin B6 (pyridoxine), vitamin B9 (folate), vitamin C (ascorbic acid), vitamin E, calcium, iron, magnesium, manganese, phosphorus, selenium and zinc.

Carrots (*Daucus carota*)

Carrots are an excellent source of antioxidant compounds and one of the richest vegetable sources of the pro-vitamin A carotenes. These antioxidant compounds help protect against cardiovascular disease, blood clots and arterial blockages, reducing the risks of heart disease. They also promote good vision, especially night vision. They can also prevent a variety of cancers and protect against the damage caused by nicotine. Eating two carrots a day can lower 'bad' LDL cholesterol by 10 per cent.

Cook or juice carrots to release nutrients from the tough cell structure to benefit from its high beta-carotene content. Research has shown that people with low levels of beta-carotene in their blood are more likely to have heart attacks and strokes and develop certain cancers. This nutrient also protects against the sun's rays. Taking carotenoids equivalent to two large carrots a day gives a natural SPF of two to four in light-skinned people.

The raw juice of parsley, carrots and celery is very valuable as nourishment for the optic system; also for the kidneys and bladder and as an aid in allaying inflammation of the urethra and genital organs.

Carrots can eliminate threadworms from children. A small cup of grated carrot taken every morning for three days, with no other food added to this meal, can clear these worms quickly.

Significant nutrients in carrots

- Carotenoids
- Fibre
- Vitamin B1 (thiamine)
- Vitamin B3 (niacin)
- Vitamin B5 (pantothenic acid)
- Vitamin B6 (pyridoxine)
- Vitamin B7 (biotin)
- Vitamin B9 (folic acid)
- Vitamin C
- Vitamin E
- Vitamin K1.

Minerals in carrots

- Boron
- Copper
- Manganese
- Molybdenum
- Potassium
- Phosphorus.

Carrots can best be grown in a container that is more than two feet deep, such as a plastic refuse bin, as carrot flies, that attack them, cannot fly higher than two feet above the ground. Cut some holes in the bottom of the bin, then add a layer of stones or broken pots for drainage. Then add sieved stone-free soil and top with a good potting compost before sowing your organic carrot seeds. Grow some spring onions around the edges to provide even more protection.

Note: Carrots, like all carotenoid-containing vegetables, should always be consumed with a fat-rich food, like avocado, olive oil, rapeseed and other plant, fish, nut or seed oils, so that the fat-soluble carotenoids can be absorbed by the body. Consuming raw carrots on their own will not provide any carotenoids to the body.

Celeriac (*Apium graveolens var. rapaceum,* celery root, German celery, knob celery, turnip rooted celery)

Celeriac is related to the carrot family and has powerful analgesic, antiallergic, antiseptic, calming and other therapeutic properties.

It can help with digestive disorders, such as constipation, diarrhoea, gastritis and indigestion, and can improve the appetite. It is also useful for arthritic pain, bladder and liver disorders, improving vision and reducing swellings.

Regular consumption of celeriac has been known to improve memory and cognitive functions and and is recommended to be eaten regularly by those with Alzheimer's disease. It is useful for those with nerve disorders, can protect the urinary system, reduce inflammation and protect against heart disease and cancers such as colon cancer and acute lymphoblastic leukaemia. Celeriac also contains nutrients that can prevent anaemia and improve bone and teeth strength.

The fact it is very low in calories (100 grams contains just 42 calories) and high in fibre and stimulates fat burning and the metabolism means celeriac is a useful food for those trying to lose weight.

Significant nutrients in celeriac

- Falcarinol
- Falcarindiol
- Fibre
- Methyl-falcarindiol
- Panaxydiol
- Vitamin A
- Vitamin B1 (thiamine)
- Vitamin B2 (riboflavin)
- Vitamin B3 (niacin)
- Vitamin B5 (pantothenic acid)
- Vitamin B6 (pyridoxine)
- Vitamin B9 (folate)

- Vitamin C
- Vitamin E
- Vitamin K1.

Minerals in celeriac

- Calcium
- Copper
- Iron
- Magnesium
- Manganese
- Phosphorus
- Potassium
- Sodium
- Zinc.

Note: People taking diuretic or anticoagulant medications should avoid celeriac. Celeriac contains some furano-coumarin compounds, such asbergapten, isopimpinellin, psoralen and xanthotoxin, which can be harmful to sensitive skin.

Chicory (*Chihorium intybus, Cichorium endivia*, escarole, common chicory, blue sailors, succory, coffee weed, cornflower, endive, radicchio, Belgian endive, French endive, red endive, sugarloaf, witloof)

Chicory is a perennial herbaceous plant of the daisy family, related to the dandelion and is native to Europe, North Africa, and Asia. Its use in herbal medicine has a long history and some of its health benefits have recently been confirmed by science. First recorded usage of it was in ancient Egypt, where it was known to have health benefits for the liver and gallbladder. Chicory is prized for the leaves, roots and buds (chicons) which are all edible. The roots are used as a tea or a caffeine-free coffee substitute and additive.

Chicory root contains inulin, which feeds the beneficial bacteria of the large intestine which in turn produce many beneficial substances, including short-chain fatty acids and certain B vitamins. They also promote further absorption of some minerals that have escaped the small intestine, including calcium and magnesium. Chicory has a mild laxative effect that is beneficial for digestive problems such as dyspepsia, indigestion and constipation.

Dried chicory roots are used to treat jaundice and as protection against liver damage. The plant contains lactucin and lactucoprin which taste bitter but can act as natural sedatives for the nervous system. A decoction of chicory root is beneficial for those with central nervous system disorders.

Chinese figwort (*Scrophularia ningpoensis*)

The Chinese figwort root has properties that can help to treat arthritis, constipation and kidney disorders. It is antibacterial, antifungal and anti-inflammatory due to its caffeic acid and flavonoid content.

Note: Avoid its use if suffering from abdominal pain, diarrhoea, dizziness or spleen or stomach disorders. It can cause bloating. It is not compatible with astragalus, Chinese dates (*Ziziphus jujube*), dogwood (*Cornus officinalis*) or ginger.

Chinese rhubarb root (*Rheum palmatum, Rheum rhaponticum, Rhizoma rhe,* false rhubarb, garden rhubarb, India rhubarb, pieplant, sweet round-leaved dock, Turkey rhubarb)

Chinese rhubarb root has been used for over two thousand years as a mild, yet effective, laxative. It supports good colon health by cleansing it and treating constipation; in smaller doses, its astringent properties ease diarrhoea and haemorrhoids. It also helps to modify the process of digestion and excretion and restore normal bodily function, acting to thoroughly cleanse and stimulate the efficient removal of waste products from the body. It not only cleanses the intestinal tract and blood, but also the liver by encouraging bile flow. It is also said to enhance and improve gallbladder function and relieve both liver and gallbladder complaints by releasing an accumulation of toxins.

As an antimicrobial, it is used to treat internal pinworms, threadworms and ringworm. The herb stimulates the uterus and is thought to move stagnated blood, which also helps to relieve pains and cramps and premenstrual tension.

Chinese rhubarb root has antibacterial, antibiotic and anti-inflammatory properties, which have made it useful for both internal and external inflammation and infection, skin eruptions, boils and carbuncles, and to promote the healing of acne, burns, cold sores, dandruff, eczema, poison ivy, poison oak, psoriasis and wounds. The anthraquinones in rhubarb can create antiviral activity against HSV I, influenza, measles and polio and it is also used for its positive effect on the mouth and nasal cavity.

Mix one teaspoon of rhubarb powder to one cup of water. Then, bring to the boil and simmer at a reduced heat for 10 minutes. Add a little honey to sweeten.

Note: Chinese rhubarb root is not recommended for long-term use and is not suitable for pregnant or breast-feeding women, children under 12 years of age, those who suffer from colitis or have intestinal obstruction or a history of renal stones or urinary problems or if taking anticoagulant (blood thinning) medicine or aspirin.

Clavo huasca (*Tynnanthus panurensis*)

The roots and stems of this Amazonian plant are macerated in aguardiente (alcohol) to make a stimulant liqueur used for rheumatism. The resin of the plant is used for fevers and toothache, being as effective as clove oil. It is also an aphrodisiac mainly for women, but reportedly excellent for males as well.

Coccinia (*Coccinia indica, Coccinia cordifolia*)

Coccinia root is used abundantly in India as it reduces inflammation in the body and has antibacterial properties which can help to treat bacterial infections. It is also a good laxative and stimulates digestion and bile production in the liver and can help to treat dysentery and parasitic infections of the intestines.

It is particularly effective at treating diabetes, orchitis and urinary tract infections.

Coccinia also helps to open pores, which can stimulate sweat, helping to eliminate toxins from the body. It is also a good wound healer and helps to treat asthma, bronchitis, colds and coughs and other respiratory disorders.

Boil chopped up coccinia roots in water for 10 to 15 minutes, strain and drink two times a day until the infection is gone.

Comfrey (*Symphytum officinale*)

Comfrey root's high concentration of mucilage makes it useful in treating stomach ulcers, inflammatory bowel disease and upper respiratory disorders. Nutrients in comfrey root nourish the pituitary gland (the master gland of the body) as well as the bones and skin and it is considered to be one of nature's great healers. It can be used to treat bronchitis, chronic coughs, diarrhoea, dysentery, glandular disorders, gout, internal ulcers and pulmonary haemorrhages, hoarseness and sore gums (as a gargle), burns (as a fomentation), fibrositis, fractures, gangrene, inflammations, mastitis, otitis, pleurisy, sores, sprains, and varicose veins. Comfrey also makes a good plant feed for vegetable and flower crops in the garden.

Cryptolepis (*Cryptolepis sanguinolenta*)

Cryptolepis is one of the top five systemic herbal antibiotics in the world and tests have found the plant to be a stronger antibacterial than the pharmaceutical antibiotic 'chloramphenicol'; this is due to the antibacterial alkaloids cryptolepine, quinoline and neocryptolepine found in this plant. They are mainly found in the root, which has been effective at treating people infected with malaria in West Africa as a decoction or tincture taken two times a day. It is also highly effective against *Candida albicans, Escherichia coli* and *Neisseria gonorrhoeae.*

Daikon (*Raphanus sativus var. longipinnatus*)

Daikon is a large mild-flavoured Asian radish eaten raw, pickled, juiced or cooked. Both the root and leaves of this brassica are edible. It can also be sprouted in a jar with a daily rinse of water. Daikon has antibacterial. anti-inflammatory, antiviral and diuretic properties. It also contains digestive enzymes that help the body process proteins, oil, fats and carbohydrates, particularly those found in raw fish. When daikon is cooked with kombu seaweed it makes a broth that removes toxins from the system. The enzymes found in daikon can counter the effects of the carcinogen nitrosamine, found in many processed foods and a few natural ones.

Raw daikon juice can also help dissolve mucus and phlegm and support the healthy function of the respiratory system. Its ability to combat bacterial and viral infections may make it an effective combatant of respiratory disease, such as bronchitis, asthma and flu. Applied topically or ingested, daikon juice has proved effective in preventing and treating acne and other skin conditions. It can also be used to cleanse the blood of toxins and support a healthy circulatory system.

Daikon radish is extremely low in fat and cholesterol, but dense in micro-nutrients, making it a great addition to the diet for the overweight or obese. These micro-nutrients include:

- vitamin B1 (thiamine)
- vitamin B2 (riboflavin)
- vitamin B3 (niacin)
- vitamin B5 (pantothenic acid)
- vitamin B6 (pyridoxine)
- vitamin B9 (folate)
- calcium
- choline
- copper
- iron
- magnesium
- manganese
- phosphorus
- potassium
- selenium
- sodium
- zinc.

These support immune function, protect against heart disease and high blood pressure, promote DNA repair and protection, and support Alzheimer's and stroke prevention and slow down the aging process.

A tea made with daikon, shittake mushrooms and kombu seaweed is used to lower fever and fight infection.

Dandelion root (*Taraxacum officinale*)

Dandelion root is a rich source of nutrients like potassium, iron and vitamins A, B, C and D. It has anti-inflammatory properties that make it effective in dealing with arthritic pain, rheumatism and other chronic joint pain conditions. It plays a vital part in reducing the level of uric acid in the body, helping to reduce pain and stiffness in the joints and increase joint mobility while relieving the symptoms of gout which arise from an excess of uric acid.

Dandelion root has natural diuretic properties that help to protect the liver and purify the blood, stimulating the removal of waste/toxins via the bile and urine while sparing the potassium that is otherwise lost with conventional diuretics. It also benefits the circulatory and glandular systems.

Commonly used as food, it is also excellent for supporting recovery from injury and surgery, has antibacterial properties that can treat many infections, including orchitis (inflammation of the testes) and urinary tract infections, and antifungal properties, especially against the *Saccharomyces cerevisiae* yeast.

Echinacea (*Echinacea purpurea, Echinacea angustifolia*, coneflower)

The chemicals contained in the root of the echinacea plant differ considerably from those in the upper part of the plant. They have high concentrations of volatile oils while the above-ground parts contain more polysaccharides which are known to trigger the activity of the immune system. They are often used in combination to shorten the duration of the common cold and flu, and reduce symptoms, such as a cough, fever and sore throat. This flower, leaf, stem and root combination can also be used to help fight infections, such as blood poisoning, diphtheria, herpes, malaria, scarlet fever, syphilis and upper respiratory and urinary tract infections as it has powerful antibacterial, antifungal and antiviral properties. It can activate the body's production of interferon, which is a specific protein that protects cells against the invasion of viruses.

Echinacea can also help to reduce the symptoms of anxiety, chronic fatigue syndrome and rheumatoid arthritis and scientific studies have validated echinacea's traditional use as a topical agent to help the body repair skin wounds and other skin problems.

Elecampane (*Lula helenium*, horse-heal, marchalan)

Elecampane roots contain volatile oils that are expectorant, anti-inflammatory and warming and can help break up congestion and calm coughs. Regular intake of elecampane root decoction can relieve symptoms of chronic bronchitis, asthma and other chronic lung conditions. Its antibacterial property is so effective that it kills the organism that causes tuberculosis. Ancient Roman healers treasured the roots of the elecampane as a digestive remedy and people have used it as a digestive stimulant and remedy for upset stomach for hundreds of years due to a chemical called alantolactone that can expel worms and parasites from the digestive tract. Taken before a meal, the root decoction has a bitter principle, called helenin, which promotes digestion, improves vitamin and mineral absorption and stimulates the appetite. This remedy is especially helpful for reviving the appetite after a bout of flu or other illness.

Elephant foot yam (*Amorphophallus paeoniifolius*, konjac root, stink lily, white spot giant arum)

The elephant foot yam is a tropical tuber crop grown mainly in Africa, South Asia, Southeast Asia and the tropical Pacific islands. It is used as a medicine and a nutritious dietary supplement. Its health benefits come from the fact that it contains 40 per cent glucomannan fibre that promotes the growth of beneficial bacteria in the colon, relieves constipation and boosts the immune system. Glucomannan has also been shown to lower blood cholesterol and help with weight loss, while improving carbohydrate metabolism. Dishes made with the elephant foot yam, such as traditional Japanese shirataki noodles, are one way to consume this nutritious root vegetable.

Fagara (*Zanthoxyloides*)

Fagara is a 'rutaceae', commonly known as the 'rue' or 'citrus' family, that is widely distributed in Uganda and other African countries and is well known for its varied uses in traditional medicine. The root-bark extract is used to treat conditions as varied as abdominal pain, elephantiasis, dysmenorrhoea, gonorrhoea, malaria, sexual impotence and toothache. Workers in West Africa have reported fagara extracts having anti-sickling (against sickle cell anaemia) and antimicrobial activity. In Nigeria fagara is used as a chewing stick; research has supported this showing antibacterial activity associated with periodontal disease. Research has also shown ethanolic extract of the root bark to have anthelmintic (antiparasitic) activity and considerable antibacterial activity effective against Lyme disease and syphilis.

False unicorn (*Chamaelirium luteum*)

The false unicorn root is considered a tonic to the reproductive organs. It also addresses symptoms of headache and depression in menopausal women. It is used for treating infertility, menstrual problems, ovarian cysts and vomiting during pregnancy. Some women take it to normalise hormones after discontinuing birth control pills.

Garlic (*Allium sativa*)

Garlic is a natural anti-inflammatory, blood thinner, cleanser and antioxidant and its historical use in cuisine and medicine dates back to 2600 BC. It is useful in the treatment of arthritis, asthma, bronchitis, cancer, colds, colitis, coughs, digestive problems, fever, flatulence, influenza, intestinal infections, lung disorders, parasitic diarrhoea, poor circulation, prostate disorders, sore throats, toothache, tumours, warts, whooping cough and yeast infections. It is also a blood purifier, detoxifies the liver, eliminates excess mucus, fights the *Toxoplasmosis gondii* parasite and protects against stomach cancers.

Garlic is capable of slowing down growth and has properties that can kill over 60 types of fungus and 20 types of bacteria, as well as some of the most potent viruses. It has now been proven scientifically that garlic is 100 times more effective than antibiotics at killing food poisoning bacteria in the intestines and does not produce the side effects of antibiotics or resistant strains of bacteria.

Garlic has been used for expelling intestinal worms and parasites by the Chinese, Greeks, Romans, Hindus and Babylonians since ancient times. It is especially useful against roundworms, giardia, trypanosome, plasmodium and leishmania. Both fresh garlic and its oil are effective.

The active components in garlic that kill parasites are allicin and ajoene. Allicin is not present in garlic until it is chopped or damaged, which is when the enzyme alliinase acts on the chemical alliin, converting it into allicin. It is therefore important to peel and chop foods from the allium family, such as chives, garlic, leeks and onions, then set them aside for 10 minutes for this process to take place before cooking or consuming. To treat parasites, finely chop or crush four cloves of garlic. allow to stand for 10 minutes, then mix with one glass of liquid (water, juice or milk) and drink daily for three weeks.

Externally, a slice of raw garlic held onto the affected skin for just a few minutes a few times a day can heal cold sores and other skin eruptions and even naturally remove cancerous moles painlessly and without surgery. Use coconut oil or vitamin E oil on the affected area afterwards. Garlic can be used externally as an infusion in oil for chest infections, earache, fungal infections, joint problems and sprains.

Garlic contains nutrients that provide nourishment for the circulatory, immune, stomach and urinary systems. It also helps to maintain normal circulation and blood pressure and to reduce cholesterol and blood fats. It is a good source of vitamins B1 (thiamine), B6 (pyridoxine), B9 (folic acid), C and K1, calcium, copper, iron, manganese, phosphorus, potassium, selenium and zinc.

Gentian root (*Gentiana lutea*)

Gentian root is one of the most useful bitter vegetable tonics with the bitter flavour stimulating the production of gastric juices to break down food and thereby stimulating the appetite. It nutritionally supports various organs, including the kidneys, liver, pancreas, spleen and stomach and is especially useful in states of exhaustion from chronic disease and in all cases of general debility and weakness. It has also been found valuable for treating jaundice.

Health disorders gentian root has been found to help

- Anaemia
- Blood impurities
- Colds
- Constipation
- Diarrhoea and dysentery
- Fever
- Gallbladder disorders
- Gout
- Flatulence
- Heart burn
- Indigestion
- Kidney disorders
- Liver disorders
- Malaria
- Menstruation (absent)
- Nausea
- Pancreas disorders
- Parasites and worms
- Poor circulation
- Spleen disorders
- Stomach cramps
- Urinary problems
- Yeast infections.

To eliminate worms and parasites take 28 grams (1 oz) of gentian root powder in a glass of any available liquid.

Note: The highly toxic white hellebore (*Veratrum album*) can be misidentified as gentian and has caused accidental poisoning when used in homemade preparations.

Ginger (*Gingiber officinalis, Zingiber officinale*)

Ginger has antioxidant, antiseptic and expectorant properties. It helps the body to eliminate wastes through the skin and increases energy. It also acts as a catalyst for other herbs, increasing their effectiveness.

Consuming 2 grams of ginger per day can produce significantly higher insulin sensitivity, which is beneficial to diabetics; it can also lower 'bad' LDL cholesterol and triglycerides. Ginger can be taken with food or as a tea and the raw peeled root can be dabbed onto the affected area for the relief of hives.

Health disorders ginger can help to treat

- Bronchitis
- Colds, coughs and influenza – helps to relieve congestion
- Digestive disorders – cleanses the digestive tract in cases of diarrhoea
- Fever – promotes perspiration
- *Helicobacter pylori* infection (and stomach ulcers)
- High blood pressure – thins blood
- Indigestion
- Menstrual cramps
- Morning sickness
- Motion sickness
- Muscle cramps
- Nausea
- Poor circulation – enhances circulation
- Sore throat.

Externally, ginger is applied as a fomentation for the treatment of pain, inflammation and stiff joints. Simmer one ounce (28 grams) of dried ginger root in two quarts (1.89 litres) of water for 10 minutes. Strain and soak a cloth in the water and apply to the affected area.

Keep changing the cloth to keep a constant warm temperature on the skin. The skin should become red as the circulation increases.

For children and adults with bronchial coughs, mix ginger root powder with a non-petroleum jelly and rub on the chest to help loosen coughs and expel mucus.

Note: Avoid cumin, ginger and turmeric if taking anticoagulants (blood thinning medication), or hormone therapies and contraceptive pills or non-steroidal anti-inflammatory medications, such as aspirin and ibuprofen, have heart problems or during the first three months of pregnancy or are breast feeding.

Ginseng (*Panax*)

The name ginseng evolved from the Chinese name meaning 'man root' derived from the root's appearance. Since the 1950s an increasing amount of worldwide research has been done that has revealed ginseng's healing properties. Nutritionally beneficial for the immune system and for long-term energy, it also has properties that can support the circulatory system and enhance mental alertness and stamina. For over 2000 years, ginseng has been used in the Far East as a tonic with revitalising properties and to help boost energy. It is especially beneficial during times of stress and fatigue because it preserves glycogen, the form of glucose that is stored in the liver and muscle cells, by increasing the use of fatty acids as a source of energy. It has been shown that the ginsenosides found in ginseng help the body to respond to stress and have endurance-enhancing effects.

Ginseng is known to have strong antibacterial, antifungal and antiviral properties, especially against the *Escherichia coli* and *Staphylococcus aureus* bacteria and the fungi *Sporothrix schenckii* and *Trichophyton rubru*.

The possibility of side effects with ginseng use is low, but high dosages may cause insomnia and nervousness.

Important note: Ginseng should be strictly avoided under the following circumstances:

- Allergic hypersensitivity
- Angina pectoris
- Asthma
- Anxiety
- Blood clotting problems
- Cardiac arrhythmia
- Children under 16 years of age
- Chronic inflammation of sexual organs
- Clotting problems
- Depression
- Emphysema
- Fibrocystic breasts
- Heart disease
- High blood pressure
- Individuals over 60 years of age
- Kidney disease
- Liver disease
- Pregnant or breast feeding women
- Prostatitis
- Schizophrenia.

Golden root (*Rhodiola rosea, Sedum roseum,* Aaron's rod, roseroot)

Golden root was used as a medicinal herb in the treatment of colds and influenza, by the Greeks, from at least 77 AD. Mongolian physicians prescribed it for cancer and tuberculosis. It is used by the Russians because of its ability to enhance work performance, eliminate fatigue and increase the capacity for exercise. It has been shown to shorten recovery time after prolonged workouts, increase attention span and enhance the memory. It can also aid weight reduction, alleviate depression, balance lung and circulatory functions, enhance the immune system, prevent high altitude sickness and strengthen the nervous system.

Golden root helps the immune system by reinstating homeostasis (metabolic balance) in the body. It also increases the natural killer cells (NK) in the stomach and spleen.

In addition, it decreases the levels of catecholamines and corticosteroids released by the adrenal glands during stress. The abnormal presence of these stress hormones can raise blood pressure, cholesterol and potassium levels, which can increase the risk of heart disease. It has also been found to decrease harmful blood lipids, thus further decreasing the risk of heart disease. It also decreases the amount of cyclic-AMP released into cardiac cells. Cyclic-AMP acts as a liaison between the outer and inner environments of the cell. It assists in the uptake of more intracellular calcium into the heart which regulates the heart beat and counteracts heart arrhythmias.

Golden seal also enhances the transport of the serotonin precursors, tryptophan and 5-hydroxytryptophan, into the brain. Serotonin is a brain neurotransmitter chemical that is involved in many functions including appetite, behaviour, blood pressure, pain perception, respiration, smooth muscle contraction and temperature regulation. When serotonin levels are correctly balanced, the brain and body will feel content and at ease. Either too much or too little serotonin has been linked to various neurological issues, including clinical depression and Parkinson's disease.

Golden root has also been reported to improve hearing, regulate blood sugar levels for diabetics and protect the liver from environmental toxins. It can also enhance thyroid function without causing hyperthyroidism, enhance thymus gland function and protect and delay involution (organ shrinkage) that occurs with aging.

Golden root can also be used to treat erectile dysfunction and premature ejaculation in men and normalises their prostatic fluid.

Goldenseal (*Hydrastis canadensis*)

American natives used goldenseal as a medication for inflammatory internal conditions such as digestive, genital, respiratory or urinary tract inflammation induced by allergy or infection. The Cherokee used the roots as a wash for external inflammations and as a decoction for general debility, dyspepsia and to improve appetite. The Iroquois used a decoction of the root for diarrhoea, fever, flatulence, liver disease, pneumonia, stomach disorders and whooping cough, and, with whiskey, for heart trouble. They also prepared a compound infusion with other roots for use as drops in the treatment of earache and as a wash for sore eyes.

Goldenseal's potent properties are primarily due to the alkaloids berberine, canadine and hydrastine which produce a powerful astringent effect on mucous membranes, reduce inflammation and have antiseptic effects. It can be used both internally and externally to help the body fight infections and soothe inflammation. This herb especially supports the glandular, liver and respiratory systems and helps cleanse the body of foreign organisms, including parasitic worms.

Henna (*Lawsonia inermis*)

The alcoholic extract of the henna root has powerful antibacterial properties due to the alkaloids and flavonoids it contains. Henna also has analgesic (pain relieving) anti-inflammatory and antipyretic (fever reducing) properties. It has been used to treat an enlarged spleen, cancer, dysentery, headaches, intestinal ulcers, liver disorders such as jaundice, and poor hair, nail and skin conditions.

Horehound root (white: *Marrubium vulgare*, black: *Ballota nigra*)

Horehound is a bitter herb from the mint family that grows like a weed in many areas of the world. Its use was first recorded in the first century AD in ancient Rome. In his manual of medicine, A. Cornelius Celsus described antiseptic uses as well as treatments for respiratory ailments using horehound juice. In his book, *On Agriculture*, first century agriculturist Lucius Columella wrote about the use of horehound for various farm animal ailments, such as ulcers, scabs and worms. In humans, it is useful for disorders of the respiratory system and acts as a natural expectorant. It can also stimulate menstrual flow and induce abortions.

Note: Excessive use of horehound root may lead to high blood pressure. It should be avoided by pregnant women.

Horse radish (*Armoracia rusticana*)

Horseradish is thought to have originated in Eastern Europe though this is uncertain. Pliny mentioned it as a medicinal herb but not as a food. It is an easy plant to grow and even a small piece of root left in the ground will produce more plants, but it does not grow well near to grapevines for reasons not yet known. If horseradish is consumed with meat it can help to protect against any bacteria that may be present within the meat.

Horseradish is a potent gastric stimulant, increases appetite and aids digestion. The volatile phytochemical compounds in the root stimulate salivary, gastric and intestinal glands to secrete digestive enzymes.

Horseradish also helps to remove harmful free radicals from the body and protect it from cancers, inflammation and infections. It has been proven in scientific studies to have powerful activity against various types of bacteria, especially those that affect the bladder, lungs, sinuses and urinary system. Take a quarter of a teaspoon of the freshly grated root and hold it in the mouth until all the taste is gone. It will immediately start loosening mucus from the sinuses to drain down the throat. This will relieve the pressure and help clear infection.

For bladder, lung, sinus and urinary system infections, mix three to four tablespoons of the fresh grated root with two tablespoons of apple cider vinegar, and honey to taste. Take the whole amount throughout the day.

Horseradish is also effective against allergies such as asthma and hay fever and acts as a diuretic.

For skin disorders, such as such as acne, blackheads, blemishes, discolorations, freckles or spots, horseradish can help as a daily skin wash.

Note: Only raw horseradish has the above medicinal properties as cooking will destroy the activity of the compounds it contains.

Horsetail (*Equisetum arvense*, common horsetail, field horsetail, shavegrass, vegetal silica)

Horsetail is an herbaceous perennial plant, native throughout the arctic and temperate regions of the northern hemisphere. Oil from the roots can be used to treat toxoplasmosis. Horsetail is also rich in 'beauty' nutrients that nourish the nails, skin, hair, bones and the body's connective tissue. It also benefits the glands and urinary tract and helps heal fractured bones because of its rich supply of nutrients. Horsetail has traditionally been used as a diuretic (helps rid the body of excess fluid by increasing urine output). Horsetail contains silica which is lethal to the eggs of parasites and so is a good remedy to eliminate worms.

Externally it can be used to stop bleeding and heal ulcers and wounds.

Note: Another species of horsetail called *Equisetum palustre* is poisonous to horses.

Ho shou wu (*Polygonum multiflorum*, flowery knotweed, fo-ti, he shou wu)

Fabled in Asian history for restoring the original colour of greying hair, compounds in the ho shou wu root can help to support the glandular, nervous and skeletal systems. This herb is also reputed to enhance the health of the liver and kidneys. The properties of ho shou wu are said to be similar to golden seal, chamomile and ginseng. It is known to help improve health, stamina and resistance to diseases. It is also effective in the prevention and treatment of neurodegenerative diseases, especially Alzheimer's disease.

Huang lian (*Coptis chinensis, Picrorhiza kurroa*)

Huang lian is a Chinese medicinal herb that has been used to treat what is now identified as type-2 diabetes for thousands of years. In 2008 it was found that the natural plant alkaloid berberine, the major active component in huang lian, is just as effective and much safer than metformin, the patent medicine most commonly now prescribed to help re-regulate blood sugar in type-2 diabetes.

Huang lian is also used for allergies, asthma, cirrhosis, fever, jaundice and liver infections caused by a virus (acute viral hepatitis). Some people use it for digestive problems, including indigestion, constipation and ongoing diarrhoea. Other uses include treatment of epilepsy, infections, malaria, rheumatoid arthritis and scorpion stings.

It is used externally to treat boils, burns, carbuncles, ear infections, eczema, painful red eyes, sore throat, toxic sores and vitiligo (a disorder that causes un-pigmented patches on the skin).

Icoja (*Unonopsis floribunda diels*)

An alcoholic maceration of the Amazonian icoja plant's root is used to treat arthritis and rheumatism, and also diarrhoea. There is another species: *Unonopsis spectabilis* also commonly called 'icoja'; its bark is used for arthritis, bronchitis, diarrhoea, lung disorders, malaria and rheumatism.

Iporuro (*Alchornea castaneifolia*)

The Amazonian Candochi-shapra and Shipibos tribes used the bark and roots of the iporuro to treat coughs and rheumatism. Others take one tablespoon of bark decoction before meals for diarrhoea. The leaves are used to increase fertility for the impotent male and it is considered to be a powerful aphrodisiac for males, sometimes found in the famous 'Rompe calzon' aphrodisiac.

Japanese or Chinese knotweed (*Fallopia japonica, Polygonum cuspidatum*)

Knotweed rhizome (part of the root) is an excellent source of the potent antioxidant resveratrol which has been shown to have positive anti-cancer and weight-loss benefits. Resveratrol helps reduce inflammation, prevents the oxidation of LDL cholesterol and makes it more difficult for platelets to stick together and form the clots that can lead to a heart attack. It is a powerful anti-aging agent and may protect nerve cells from damage and the build-up of neurofibrillary tangles in the brain that are associated with Alzheimer's disease.

Resveratrol also helps prevent insulin resistance, a condition in which the body becomes less sensitive to the effects of the blood sugar-lowering hormone, insulin, and which can lead to type-2 diabetes. Knotweed root is also known to kill the bacterium responsible for Lyme disease.

Note: Avoid Chinese or Japanese knotweed if pregnant or taking anticoagulants (blood thinning medications) or non-steroidal anti-inflammatory drugs such as aspirin and ibuprofen, due to the risk of bleeding.

Jergon sacha (*Dracontium loretense*)

The root of the Amazonian jergon sacha tree is used to treat snakebites. Indigenous people repel snakes by whipping their feet and legs with the branches. The corms/roots can also be used to control and steady the shaking hands of Parkinson's disease. It also has very powerful antiviral and antibacterial properties and is especially useful in fighting HIV/AIDS and cancer (taken together with cat's claw and/or pau d'arco).

Jerusalem artichoke (*Helianthus tuberosus*, earth apple, sunchoke, sun root, topinambour)

The Jerusalem artichoke, not to be confused with the globe artichoke (*Cynara scolymus*), is the tuber of a species of sunflower native to eastern North America. It has no relation to Jerusalem and it is not even a type of artichoke, though both are members of the daisy family.

The Jerusalem artichoke is rich in the carbohydrate inulin (76 per cent), which is a polymer of the monosaccharide fructose. Inulin contains fructans, which are food for beneficial bacteria in the gut, but if the tubers are stored for any length of time, they will digest the inulin into its component fructose (fruit sugar). Inulin (not to be confused with the hormone insulin) is a zero-calorie, saccharine, and inert carbohydrate, which does not metabolise inside the human body, and therefore, make this tuber an ideal sweetener for diabetics and dieters when consumed fresh. It is an especially good addition to soups.

Jerusalem artichokes contain 10 per cent protein which is more than most other root vegetables and are particularly high in the sulphur-containing essential amino acids cysteine, homocysteine, methionine and taurine. These components are essential for maintaining the flexibility of connective tissue as well as helping the liver carry out detoxification, which helps protect against cancer and hepatitis.

Jerusalem artichokes also promote regular bowel movements, which protects against bowel cancer. Regular consumption can lower blood pressure, LDL cholesterol and triglyceride levels due to their rich potassium content, and prevent anaemia due to their high iron content. They contain 650 milligrams of potassium per 150 grams. They also contain vitamin B1 (thiamine), vitamin B3 (niacin), phosphorus and copper.

Jicama (*Pachyrhizus erosus*, Mexican turnip, Mexican yam)

Jicama, also known as the Mexican turnip or yam, is a root vegetable similar to the sweet potato. It has been consumed as a vegetable and used medicinally in Central and South America for thousands of years. It is most commonly eaten raw seasoned with spices like chilli and fruit juices. It can be cooked but this will reduce some of its powerful health benefits.

Regular consumption of jicama can boost brain function and the immune system, build strong bones, help to manage diabetes, improve circulation and digestion, increase energy levels, lower blood pressure, prevent various types of cancer and heart disease and help with weight management.

The jicama tuber is a rich source of dietary fibre, copper, iron, magnesium, manganese, potassium and vitamins B2, B5, B6, B9, C and E.

Note: The tubers are highly nutritious but all other components of the plant (including the seeds) are poisonous.

Kava kava (*Piper methysticum*)

Kava kava's botanical name roughly translated means 'intoxicating pepper'. The rhizome (underground stem) is used as a sedative to alleviate stress, anxiety and insomnia and soothe the nerves. The active components in kava root are called kavalactones. Specific types of kavalactones include dihydrokavain, methysticin, kavain, dihydromethysticin, dihydrokawain, yangonin and desmethoxyyangonin.

Note: Possible side effects of over consumption of kava can include drowsiness, headaches, indigestion, mouth numbness, rash and visual disturbances. Chronic or heavy use of kava has been linked to blood abnormalities, kidney damage, loss of muscle control, pulmonary hypertension and skin scaling. Kava may also lower blood pressure and interfere with blood clotting, so it should not be used by people with bleeding disorders. People with Parkinson's disease should avoid kava because it may worsen symptoms and it should not be taken within two weeks of surgery. Pregnant and nursing women, children and people with liver or kidney disease should also avoid it.

Kudzu root (*Pueraria lobatam*, Japanese arrowroot)

A relative to the pea family and native to China (known as gé gēn) and Japan, kudzu is a voracious invasive plant that is often sprayed with herbicide so the source is important. It contains the isoflavones puerarin and daidzein (an anti-inflammatory and antimicrobial agent) and daidzin (structurally related to genistein). Kudzu root can combat both gram-negative and gram-positive food-borne pathogens in various foods, especially liquid foods.

It can help to relieve headaches and migraines and is often used for allergies and diarrhoea. In Chinese medicine, it is considered one of the 50 fundamental herbs and is used to treat alcoholism, hangovers, tinnitus and vertigo. Kudzu may also be helpful in treating Alzheimer's disease, cardiovascular disease and diabetes. The roots, flowers and leaves of kudzu all show antioxidant activity.

Lady's slipper (*Cypripedium areitinum, Cypripedium calceolus, Cypripedium pubescens*, American valerian, bleeding heart, moccasin flower, monkey flower, nerve root, Noah's ark, orchid, slipper root, venus shoe, yellows)

Lady's slipper is a member of the orchid family and its root has many nerve-calming properties. The plant was held in high regard by the indigenous tribes of America who used it to ease menstrual and labour pains and to counter insomnia and nervous conditions, headaches, spasms and cramps. The Chippewa placed the dried and remoistened root directly onto skin inflammations and toothaches to relieve discomfort. The Cherokee used one variety to treat worms in children. It has also been used to treat chorea, depression, headaches, hypochondria, hysteria, insomnia, low fevers, nervous unrest, reflex function disorders and stomach disorders.

Like valerian (page 106) but even more so, lady's slipper is an effective tranquilliser, reducing emotional tension and promoting sleep. However, because of its scarcity and cost, lady's slipper is now used only on a small scale as a sedative and for relaxing such stress-related disorders as palpitations, headaches, muscular tension, panic attacks and neurotic conditions.

Land caltrop (*Tribulus terrestris*, abrojos, al gutub, bai ji li, gokshura, puncture vine, tack weed)

The fruit, leaves and roots of land caltrop have properties known to optimise the function of the prostate and urinary tract and can help to treat orchitis, which is a swelling of one or both testicles. It contains a saponin which is also known to help with premature ejaculation and sexual function by increasing sperm production, motility, survival time and the quality of the sperm. It can also help to treat the andropause in men, urinary tract infections and dysuria (painful urination) associated with cystitis. It is a diuretic herb.

It has properties which can help to support the liver and kidneys and to treat anaemia, diabetes, high blood pressure and high cholesterol levels. It also helps to strengthen and enhance the blood circulation and immune system. If taken with ginger it can help to treat gout. It also promotes a good mood and helps to counteracts anxiety, depression, nervousness and stress.

To treat bladder and kidney stones, make a paste with land caltrops seed powder and mix with honey. Take one teaspoon three times a day until the stones are gone.

It also helps to promote recovery after physical exertion and is popular with athletes.

Note: Land caltrop can cause miscarriage and must be avoided by pregnant or breast feeding women or individuals with breast or prostate cancer. Excess consumption of land caltrop can cause sleep disturbances and irregular menstruation, and high doses may adversely affect the eyes and liver.

Liquorice root (*Glycyrrhiza glabra*)

Liquorice root nutritionally supports the respiratory and gastrointestinal systems, heart and spleen. It can soothe irritated mucous membranes and help the body get rid of unwanted mucus with its expectorant properties. Liquorice root has properties similar to cortisone and oestrogen. It stimulates the adrenal glands and helps the body cope with stress.

Genuine liquorice root has been a key ingredient in most Chinese herbal formulas for more than 3000 years. Research indicates that liquorice's two primary ingredients - glycyrrhizin and glycyrrhetinic acid - boost production of interferon. Active ingredients hypericin and pseudohypericin, display sufficiently strong antiviral properties to overpower *Herpes simplex* viruses type 1 and 2, certain flu viruses (influenza A and B) and Epstein Barr virus (EBV).

It can also treat chronic hepatitis B. Glycyrrhizin interferes with hepatitis B surface antigen and is synergistic with interferon against hepatitis A virus. It is also used at times to treat hepatitis C. Liquorice root helps protect the liver from damage from chemotherapy. At low doses, the herb stimulates the liver to manufacture cholesterol and excrete it in bile. This can help lower serum cholesterol levels.

Note: If suffering from high blood pressure, a heart condition, oedema or taking certain medications such as warfarin or diuretics, do not take liquorice root.

Mandrake (*Mandragora officianarum, Atropa mandragora*, Alraun, Devil's testicles, Mandragora, Satan's apple)

The Greek word 'Mandragora', from which mandrake is derived, implies a plant that is harmful to cattle, which indeed it is. Extracts from the mandrake root can support the liver, gallbladder and all aspects of digestion and can exert a powerful and beneficial influence on the glands but care must be taken with preparation as it is a poisonous plant for most mammals, including humans, and therefore it should only be consumed with the advice of an experienced herbalist.

Note: Mandrake contains the tropane alkaloid phytochemicals atropine, cuscohygrine, hyoscyamine, mandragorine and scopolamine that have a powerful effect on the central nervous system; extreme caution is therefore advised. The 'apples' are narcotic, milder than the root, but still powerful enough to kill if taken in excessive quantity.

Marshmallow (*Althea officinalis*, altea, ghasul, hatmi, iviscus, khitmi, khatmah, mallow, umalvavisco, subeni-tati-aoi, white mallow)

The marshmallow herb should not be confused with the confectionery of the same name. This is a herb native to Europe which thrives in an environment of dark and salty marshes. Its botanical name '*Althainein*', means 'to heal' and the root is the part that is mostly used for this purpose. It is dug up in the late autumn, cleaned of fibres and then shredded or desiccated immediately.

Marshmallow root has soothing properties and nutritionally supports the respiratory and gastrointestinal systems. It has a long history dating back thousands of years as an herbal remedy for cough, sore throat and other respiratory problems such as bronchitis and whooping cough (pertussis). This is due to the large amounts of mucilage found in the root and also the flower. This forms a protective coating to soothe tissues that have become inflamed and irritated. This coating protects the digestive and urinary tract when kidney stones pass. A daily intake of two pints (1.1 litres) of marshmallow root tea can effectively flush out kidney stones from the body.

Other important consituents, especially of the leaves and roots, are polysaccharides with antibacterial properties that are especially effective against the *Escherichia coli* and *Klebsiella pneumoniae* strains of bacteria. A syrup made from the roots is good for treating bronchitis, laryngitis and respiratory or urinary system infections. Thanks to the mucilage content, it is also good for healing a leaky gut which can prevent autoimmune reactions and can help to treat inflammatory disorders such as irritable bowel syndrome and ulcerative colitis.

Health problems marshmallow can be used to remedy

- Bronchitis
- Colitis
- Crohn's disease
- Diarrhoea

- Enteritis
- Excess stomach acid
- Gastritis
- Gastroesophageal reflux disease (GERD)
- Hiatus hernia
- Indigestion
- Inflammation and irritation of the urinary and respiratory mucous linings
- Irritable bowel syndrome (IBS)
- Kidney stones
- Mouth ulcers
- Peptic ulcers
- Ulcerative colitis (IBD)
- Whooping cough (pertussis).

As a mouthwash and anti-cough and respiratory agent, two grams (0.07 ounces) of the root should be put into one cup (237 ml) of cold water and soaked for two hours and the water then gargled with. A tea made from the roots may also be used as a mouthwash and to treat inflammation and mouth ulcers. The root may also be peeled fresh and given to infants to chew on for teething issues. See *Nature Cures For Babies*.

External uses

Externally, shredded root should be mixed with enough warm water to form a thick paste and spread onto a clean cloth. Apply to irritated areas as needed. It can then be used to treat:

- Cuts, scrapes and other wounds
- Dislocations
- Eczema
- Bruises
- Insect bites

- Painful muscles
- Pink eye
- Psoriasis
- Skin inflammations
- Splinters.

Note: Caution should be taken by those suffering from alcohol dependency, diabetes or liver disorders. Use is not recommended for pregnant or breastfeeding women.

Marsh marica (*Cipura paludosa*)

The marsh marica is very common on sea beaches and in coastal marshes. Research has shown that ethanolic extract (see Tinctures, page 9) from bulbs of this plant can reduce long-lasting learning and memory deficits induced by prenatal methylmercury exposure in mice but this preparation has not been tried on humans yet and very little information can be found about it.

Mashua (*Tropaeolum tuberosum*, añu, cubio, isanu, puel, ysaño)

The mashua is a perennial climbing tuber/salad crop from the Andes related to the nasturtium. It has been cultivated since approximately 5500 BC and is an important food source for more than nine million indigenous people living in the Andes mountains at elevations between 2500 and 4000 meters. One plant can yield up to 4 kilos of tubers. This, plus the ease of cultivation, makes it a good crop to grow for both human and animal consumption. Both the tubers and vigorous profusion of leaves are edible. The tubers contain isothiocyanates (mustard oils) that give them a sharp, peppery taste reminiscent of hot radishes when eaten raw. When cooked, they turn sweet.

Mashua is resistant to many insects, nematodes (parasitic worms), fungi and other pathogens, including the Andean weevil which attacks potatoes and other tuber crops. These insect repellent properties make it a very good companion plant but cabbage white butterflies are strongly attracted so it is best planted where birds can easily feast on caterpillars.

The tuber has antibiotic and diuretic properties and can treat nephropathy (damage or disease of the kidneys), eliminate bladder and kidney stones, treat skin ulcers and kill lice. It also has an-aphrodisiac effects and was used by the Incas to feed troops to keep their minds on fighting as it causes a drop in the levels of testosterone/dihydrotestosterone. In Bolivia, it is used to induce menstruation as it has a beneficial effect on oestrogen in females. It has also been shown to prevent the development of cancerous cells in the stomach, colon, prostate and skin.

Note: Mashua must be consumed with fatty foods like avocado, nut, seed, olive or fish oils in order to absorb the fat-soluble carotenoids it contains.

Moringa (*Moringa oleifera*, ben oil tree, benzoil tree, drumstick tree, horseradish tree)

Moringa is a tree native to parts of Africa and Asia. Its name is derived from murungai/muringa, the Tamil/Malayalam word for drumstick. The leaves and seeds are most often used for medicine but the roots and bark have more powerful concentrations of the same components that can be used medicinally so care must be taken. The roots and bark are used for cardiac and circulatory problems, as a tonic and for inflammation.

The alkaloid spirachin (a nerve paralyser) has been found in the roots and the gum has diuretic, astringent (a drying, tightening effect on tissues to aid wound healing) and abortifacient (causes miscarriage) properties and is also used to treat asthma.

In Senegal and India, moringa roots are pounded and mixed with salt to make a poultice for treating rheumatism and joint pains. In Senegal, this poultice is also used to relieve lower back or kidney pain.

Note: Pregnant women should be aware of moringa's ability to induce miscarriage.

Disorders moringa can help to remedy and protect against

- Anaemia
- Anxiety
- Asthma

- Arthritis
- Bacterial infections
- Boils

- Bone disorders
- Bronchitis
- Cancer
- Cholera
- Colds
- Colitis
- Cramp
- Cystitis
- Depression
- Diabetes type-2
- Diarrhoea
- Digestive disorders
- Dysentery
- Ear infections
- Epilepsy
- Erectile dysfunction
- Eye infections
- Fungal and yeast infections
- Gout
- Heart problems
- High blood pressure
- Hysteria
- Inflammation
- Joint disorders
- Liver disorders
- Malnutrition
- Obesity
- Orchitis
- Parasites and worms
- Poor circulation
- Prostate disorders
- Respiratory disorders
- Rheumatism
- Sexually transmitted diseases
- Scurvy
- Skin disorders
- Sleep disorders
- Spleen disorders
- Stomach ulcers
- Throat infections
- Tuberculosis
- Urinary disorders
- Urinary tract infection
- Varicose veins
- Water retention.

Mucura (*Petiveria alliacea*, anamu, apacin, apacina, apazote de zorro, aposin, ave, aveterinaryte, calauchin, chasser vermine, congo root, douvant-douvant, emeruaiuma, garlic weed, guinea henweed, guine, guinea, guinea hen leaf, gully root, herbe aux poules, hierba de las gallinitas, huevo de gato, kojo root, kuan, kudjuruk, lemtewei, lemuru, mal pouri, mapurit, mapurite, mucura-caa, mucura, mucuracáa, ocano, payche, pipi, tipi, verbena hedionda, verveine puante, zorrillo)

Mucura is an Amazonian plant that is a strong immune system enhancer as well as a powerful pain killer. It contains compounds that increase the actions of the body's immune cells which are responsible for tracking down and removing foreign cells like bacteria and cancer. It also has broad-spectrum antimicrobial properties against a wide variety of bacteria, fungi, viruses and yeasts, including *Candida albicans*, *Escherichia coli*, *Mycobacterium tuberculosis*, *Pseudomonas*, *Shigella* and *Staphylococcus*.

Mucura contains benzaldehyde and coumarin, both of which have anticancer properties. It is also an excellent remedy for hip and knee osteoarthritis and severe arthritis and is anti-inflammatory for treating gastritis and gout. It has been used to stimulate growth in children and teenagers and is also known to help support the thymus gland. It is also good for caring for the veins and blood circulation and helping to treat vascular diseases.

Properties of mucura

- Abortifacient (induces abortions)
- A memory enhancer
- Analgesic (pain reliever)
- Anti-spasmodic (relieves involuntary spasms of muscles)
- Anti-pyretic (prevents or reduces fever)
- Anti-rheumatic
- Contraceptive
- Diuretic (increases the production of urine)
- Emmenagogue (stimulates and increases menstrual flow)
- Mental stimulant
- Sudorific (induces sweating)
- Vermifuge (kills and expels parasites).

Onion (*Allium cepa*)

Regular consumption of onions can help to prevent cancer, circulatory disorders and heart disease. They are particularly useful in reducing the development of bladder cancer in smokers. Onions contain vitamin C, vitamin K1, vitamin B9 (folic acid), chromium, quercetin and allicin.

As with chives, garlic and leeks, onions should always be

left to stand for 10 minutes after chopping, before cooking or eating, to allow the production of allicin to take place. Allicin is a phytochemical with powerful antimicrobial and tumour-fighting properties. It can also help to reduce atherosclerosis and fat deposition and normalise the lipoprotein balance, plus decrease blood pressure. It has anti-thrombotic and anti-inflammatory activities and functions as an antioxidant.

Oregon grape root (*Berberis aquifolium, Berberis vulgaris, Berberis aristata, Tinospora cordifolia*)

Oregon grape root is a rich source of berberine, a compound that is highly effective against bacteria, fungi, parasites, protozoa, viruses and worms. Berberine is an isoquinoline alkaloid present in the roots, rhizome and stem bark of this plant. The potential importance of berberine is indicated by its use in the Indian Ayurvedic, Unani and Chinese systems of medicine.

Berberine has potent anti-arrhythmic (corrects an abnormal heart rate), anti-diarrhoeal and anti-tumour activities. It has been shown in studies to inhibit the proliferation of oesophageal cancer cells and cyclooxygenase-2 transcriptional activity in human colon cancer cells.

In 2008 it was also discovered that berberine is just as effective and much safer than metformin, the medicine most commonly now prescribed to help re-regulate blood sugar in type-2 diabetes.

Parsnips (*Pastinaca sativa*)

Parsnips contain far more heart-friendly potassium and vitamin B9 (folate) than carrots. Folate is required for the creation of healthy cells and having insufficient levels of it has been linked to cancer and birth defects. Parsnips are a good source of choline, falcarinol, falcarindiol, panaxydiol, methyl-falcarindiol, vitamin B1, vitamin B3, vitamin B5, vitamin B6, vitamin B9, vitamin C (17% of RDA), vitamin E, calcium, copper, iron, potassium, manganese and phosphorus. Manganese helps nourish the nerves and brain and assists the coordination of nerve impulses and muscular actions. It also helps eliminate fatigue and reduces nervous irritability.

Parsnips are a rich source of both soluble and insoluble dietary fibre; 100 grams of parsnips provides 4.9 grams compared with potatoes, which contain only 2.2 grams per 100 grams. It is recommended that an average-sized adult should consume around 25 grams of fibre per day and this will then help to reduce blood cholesterol levels and lower the risk of heart attacks and strokes. It will also help to fight obesity and stop constipation and other digestive and excretory issues from occurring. Parsnips can be cooked and prepared in the same way as potatoes (baked, boiled, roasted, steamed and mashed) as a sweet-tasting alternative.

One hundred grams of cooked parsnips contains only 55 calories. In Europe, parsnips were used to sweeten jams and cakes before sugar was widely available and helped the jam to set, making them a good alternative to sugar.

Pepperwort (*Lepidium meyenii*, ayak chichira, ayuk willku, ginseng andin, ginseng Péruvien, lepidium peruvianum, maca maca, maca Péruvien, maino, maka, Peruvian ginseng, Peruvian maca, maca root, peppergrass)

Pepperwort is a plant that grows in central Peru in the Andes mountains. It has been cultivated as a vegetable crop here since at least 1600 BC and is a staple food of the indigenous people in this region to this day due to its very rich nutritional content. It is a brassica related to radish, mustard and cress, with an odour similar to butterscotch. Its root is used to make medicine. It can also be baked and used as a vegetable like sweet potato.

Pepperwort is rich in sugars, protein, starches and essential micronutrients. It contains alkaloids, whole fibre, lipids, 20 amino acids, beta-ecdysone, beta-sitosterol, hydrolyzable carbohydrates, fatty acids (including linolenic, palmitic and oleic acids), glucosinolates, isothiocyanates, iodine, phosphorus, potassium, iron, magnesium, zinc, calcium, steroid glycosides, saponins, sitosterols, stigmasterol, tannins, and vitamins B1, B2, B12, C and E.

The glucosinolates found in the root help to combat serious invasive infection and are said to be particularly effective in building the body's defences against serious malignant illnesses.

Pepperwort is used medicinally to treat anaemia, chronic fatigue syndrome, constipation, depression and hypothyroidism and to boost the immune system. It is also used to treat HIV/

AIDS, leukaemia, stomach cancer and tuberculosis. It has properties which can improve bone density and can be very helpful for those suffering from osteoporosis.

It is also useful for treating hormone imbalances, menstrual problems and symptoms of menopause and erectile dysfunction and can improve fertility and sexual health due to the compounds that can balance the sex hormones. It has a reputation for being a powerful aphrodisiac and, as it is rich in minerals like zinc and iodine and essential fatty acids, it can improve mood and overall brain health.

Because it is rich in essential fatty acids, minerals, protein and vitamins, pepperwort is known to improve sports performance and provides faster repair from sports injuries. It can enhance athletic performance, energy, memory, mental clarity and stamina.

Piri piri root (*Cyperus articulatus*)

The root of this Amazonian plant can help treat influenza and has febrifuge (reduces fever), haemostatic (stops bleeding) and vulnerary (heals wounds) properties. It can also treat snake bites and is an abortifacient (induces abortion).

Plantain (*Plantago lancelota, Plantago major, Plantago ovato*)

Plantain root has wide-ranging antimicrobial properties besides being anti-inflammatory and analgesic. A decoction is used in the treatment of a wide range of complaints, including asthma, bronchitis, catarrh, coughs, cystitis, diarrhoea, dysentery, gastritis, hay fever, irritable bowel syndrome, haemorrhoids, peptic ulcers and sinusitis. It is a safe and effective treatment for bleeding as it quickly stops blood flow and encourages the repair of damaged tissue without scarring. The active biochemical aucubin is mainly responsible for the antimicrobial action of this plant.

Note: Plantain can cause allergic skin reactions so should be tested on a small area first. If taken internally it may cause diarrhoea and low blood pressure.

Poke root (*Phytolacca americana, Phytolacca decandra*, American nightshade, bear's grape, ink berry, pigeon berry, poke berry, poke bush, poke sallet, poke weed, red weed, Virginia poke)

The botanical name of the poke bush comes from the Greek word φυτόν (phyton), meaning 'plant' and the Latin word 'lacca', a red dye. It has antiarthritic, antibacterial, anti-inflammatory, anti-rheumatic and antiviral properties and is also very effective in treating lymphatic disorders and boosting the immune system. It is also known to treat various types of skin disorder, fungal infections like ringworm and scabies, and eye infections such as conjunctivitis.

Decoctions made from poke root can also treat catarrh, constipation, dysmenorrhoea, dyspepsia, Lyme disease, mumps, pharyngitis, respiratory infections, sore throats, syphilis and tonsillitis.

It may also be helpful in treating diseases related to the immune system, such as HIV/AIDS, as it has certain properties that help strengthen the immune system by interacting with the proliferating T-cells. It also has potential to help treat breast and uterine cancers and is known to shrink tumours. Poke root extracts are also used as insect repellents and are considered to be extremely effective.

Poke root contains, among many important components, glycoproteins, resins, tannins, triterpene saponins, and an active glycoprotein lectin called pokeweed mitogen which stimulates lymphocytes.

Important note: The whole of the plant is toxic and increases in toxicity through the year, with children being at particular risk from its very poisonous purple-red ripe fruit. The juice of poke root can be absorbed through the skin and therefore contact of plant parts with bare skin should be avoided. Care must be taken to prepare it properly when using this herb medicinally.

Potato (*Solanum tuberosum*)

The potato belongs to the *Solanaceae* or nightshade family whose other members include aubergines, goji berries, peppers and tomatoes. Potatoes originated in the Andean mountain region of South America and have been cultivated by the Indians living in these areas for between 4000 and 7000 years. Unlike many other foods, potatoes can be grown at the high altitudes typical of this area and therefore became a staple food for these hardy people. Potatoes were brought to Europe by Spanish explorers who 'discovered' them in South America in the early 16th century.

Since potatoes are a good source of vitamin C, they were subsequently used on Spanish ships to prevent scurvy. They were introduced into Europe via Spain, and while they were consumed by some people in Italy and Germany, initially they were not widely consumed throughout Europe, even though many governments actively promoted this nutritious foodstuff that was relatively inexpensive to produce. The reason for this is that since people knew that the potato was part of the nightshade family, many felt that it must be poisonous like some of its relations. In addition, many regarded potatoes with suspicion since they were not mentioned in the Bible. In fact, potatoes initially had such a poor reputation in Europe that many people thought eating them would cause leprosy.

Potatoes are useful for easing indigestion, colic, gastritis, ulcers and constipation. Externally, they are useful for minor burns, sunburn, inflamed skin, skin infections, chilblains and even headaches.

They are a good source of fibre, carbohydrates, asparagine, caffeic acid, carotenoids, flavonoids, quercetin, kukoamines, patatin, tryptophan, vitamin B1 (thiamine), vitamin B5 (pantothenic acid), vitamin B6 (pyridoxine), vitamin B9 (folic acid), vitamin C, copper, potassium and manganese.

New potatoes are also a source of potassium and vitamin

C is highest in freshly harvested new potatoes. All potatoes are low in sugar, virtually fat free and very low in sodium and are around 100 calories less than the same-sized serving of white rice or pasta. They are best baked and consumed with the skins to preserve and concentrate all the nutrients.

White potatoes that have turned green and potato leaves contain a compound called solanine which is poisonous. Solanine is a steroid glycoside of the saponin group found in plants from the nightshade family, which, in large doses, can cause gastrointestinal disorders such as diarrhoea and vomiting, hallucinations, paralysis and even death.

One of the triggers for solanine to develop in a white potato is exposure to light, especially fluorescent light. Therefore, it is essential to store potatoes in a dark place, preferably between 10°C (50°F) and 18°C (65°F). If potatoes must be stored in a lighted place, they can be kept in a brown paper bag loosely closed to allow for air circulation.

Cooked potatoes are not a concern when it comes to acrylamide, a potentially toxic and cancer-causing substance that is produced by heating asparagine. However, fried, processed foods made with potatoes, such as potato chips and French fries, are considered among the highest risk of foods when it comes to acrylamide exposure. This is a reason to avoid or minimise intake of these foods.

Note: Potatoes are among the 12 foods on which pesticide residues have been most frequently found. Therefore, individuals wanting to avoid pesticide-associated health risks may want to avoid consumption of potatoes unless they are grown organically.

Queen of the meadow (*Filipendula ulmaria, Spiraea ulmaria*, bridewort, gravel root, gravel weed, meadowsweet, meadow wort, meadwort, quaker lady, trumpet weed)

Queen of the meadow has been used historically since the herbalist Thomas Culpepper's time to treat colds, coughs, headaches and flu. It has antacid, astringent, anti-inflammatory, antirheumatic, carminative (antiflatulence), diaphoretic (induces perspiration), diuretic (stimulates urine production), antiemetic (reduces nausea and vomiting) and stomachic (stimulates the appetite) properties and the root is traditionally valued to help heal strains, sprains, and the associated aches. It nourishes the ligaments and tendons and assists in restoring their normal function and so is useful and effective for treating arthritis. Taken as a decoction, it helps release inorganic deposits from the joints and tissues and can prevent some types of bladder stones.

Quisqualis indica (*Combretum indicum*, Chinese honeysuckle, rangoon creeper)

Quisqualis indica is a vine with red flower clusters found in Asia. The genus translates into Latin for 'What is that?' Decoctions of the root, seed or fruit can be used as an anthelmintic to expel parasitic worms or to alleviate diarrhoea. The roots are also used to treat rheumatism.

Radishes (*Raphanus sativus*)

Radishes belong to the brassica family and can be white, red, purple or black, long, cylindrical or spherical in shape. They are eaten raw, cooked or pickled. Radish is also known as daikon (see page 36) in some parts of the world. Radishes may be considered under the general classification of either large or small. The large contain a little more than 85% water, but 50% less mineral elements than the small. The small radishes are used either whole or sliced to garnish salads, while the large radishes can be grated or shredded as an ingredient.

Radishes contain a volatile ether which is particularly useful as a solvent for mucus or phlegm. They also contain enzymes valuable in aiding the secretion of digestive juices. Because of their diuretic action, they are valuable in cleansing the kidneys and the bladder. The juice of radishes blended with carrot juice is a wonderful aid in cleansing and healing the mucous membrane of the digestive system as well as of the respiratory organs.

Radish is good for the liver and as a detoxifier to purify the blood. It is very useful for treating jaundice as it helps remove bilirubin and checks its production. It also checks destruction of red blood cells during jaundice by increasing the supply of fresh oxygen in the blood. The black radish and the leaves are best for this purpose.

Regular consumption of radishes can help to relieve and remedy asthma, bronchitis, constipation, fever, gall bladder, kidney and liver disorders, haemorrhoids (piles), respiratory disorders, urinary infections, skin disorders and many forms of cancer. They are also useful for weight loss and can be used externally for insect bites.

Radishes are low in saturated fat and very low in cholesterol, a good source of vitamin B2 (riboflavin), vitamin B6 (pyridoxine), calcium, copper, magnesium, manganese and phosphorus and a very rich source of chlorine, dietary fibre, vitamin B9 (folate), vitamin C and potassium, silicon, sodium and sulphur.

Rampion (*Campanula rapunculus*)

The word 'rampion' means bellflower and is derived from its Latin specific name, *rapunculus* that comes from 'rapa' (turnip). It is a garden vegetable originating from Asia, Europe and North Africa and possesses roots that are similar to turnips that can be boiled tender, like parsnips. The rampion root can be used as a vegetable for soups and as an accompaniment to meat dishes or raw in salads. It contains inulin, a sugar substitute, and it is often used in special dietary foods for diabetics. It also contains calcium, iron, phosphorus, mucilage, cellulose, rubber resin, choline and mineral salts. Rampion has anti-inflammatory benefits, which have been known to help create a calmer pregnancy and more successful birth. It has also been used to treat angina.

Reed mace (*Typha latifolia variegata*)

Evidence of preserved starch grains on grinding stones suggests reed mace was eaten in Europe 30,000 years ago. The boiled root stock can be used as a diuretic for increasing urination. The cooked root can be used mashed to make a jelly-like poultice for boils, burns, scabs, sores and wounds.

Restharrow (*Ononis repens*)

The common restharrow is a perennial member of the pea family found by the sea shore and in dry hill pastures in chalk or limestone areas. It is a favourite food of the donkey, from which the generic name is derived, 'onos' - the Greek word for an ass. A tradition exists that this was the plant from which the crown of thorns was plaited for the Crucifixion.

Restharrow is a good source of calcium, iron, magnesium and sulphur. It also possesses aperient (relieves constipation), diuretic (stimulates urine production), expectorant (loosens phlegm), metabolic stimulant (increases energy) and sedative (aids sleep) properties. It is good for treating oedema and water retention, especially uric acid retention, gravel and stones (see next). It is also recommended for urinary mucus, kidney inflammation and rheumatism. A decoction of the roots can also be used externally for eczema, itching and other skin problems.

The sweet viscid juice extracted from the root can be used to treat toxoplasmosis, bladder stones and delirium.

To make an infusion, steep three to four tablespoons of chopped roots in one cup of hot water for five minutes while stirring. Take one, to one and a half, cups per day, warm.

To make a decoction, soak two teaspoons of the chopped roots in half a cup of cold water for eight hours, then bring rapidly to the boil. Simmer for 10 minutes, then cool and strain. Drink once a day for one week. The decoction can also be added to sauces, soups and teas.

Salsify (*Tragopogon porrifolius*, goat's beard, oyster plant, vegetable oyster)

Salsify is a vegetable whose roots and leaves can be cooked. It is a member of the sunflower family and its varieties are named 'French Blue Flowered' and the 'Mammoth Sandwich Island'. It is cultivated in Asia (Taiwan), Central and Southern Europe and the United States and is said to have originated in the Mediterranean.

Salsify contains no cholesterol or fat and is low in sodium. It is an excellent source of dietary fibre, inulin, vitamin A (retinol), vitamin B9 (folate), vitamin C, calcium, phosphorus, potassium and magnesium.

Sarsaparilla (*Smilax longifolia*)

Sarsaparilla is an Amazonian plant used in cases of pruritus and erythema (redness of skin). There is another plant commonly called 'zarzaparilla' (*Smilax regelii*) and the roots are mainly used in decoctions and infusions as anti-inflammatory, antirheumatic, ant-flu and anti-syphilitic. Sarsaparilla was discovered by the early Spanish settlers in Jamaica, Peru, St Domingo and Brazil in the middle of the 16th century. It was introduced into Seville about 1536 from 'New Spain' and another variety soon arrived from Honduras. Pedro de Cieze de Leon in 1553 wrote that he saw it growing in South America. It was recommended as a cure for syphilis and for some time was considered the only effective remedy for this ailment. It was from the time of its introduction considered a superior blood purifier. It fell into disuse for a while until Sir William Fordyce revived it in 1757. After this short resurgence, it was again ignored. During the latter part of the 19th century its use was considered the result of ignorant superstition. In 1928, however, Perutz studied it extensively and concluded that it really did help in the treatment of syphilis, probably by stimulating the body's defensive mechanism; it may also be effective against the Lyme disease bacterium.

Sarsaparilla also possesses the following properties: alterative (restores proper functions of the body), aphrodisiac (stimulates sexual desire), antibiotic, anti-inflammatory, antirheumatic, antiseptic, carminative (relieves flatulence), depurative (detoxifying), diaphoretic (induces perspiration), diuretic (stimulates urine production), febrifuge (reduces fever), formonal (balances hormones), protects the liver against hepatitis, steroidal (anti-inflammatory), stimulant, stomachic (stimulates appetite) and a tonic. It also contains substances which are similar to the male hormone testosterone and the female hormone progesterone and it can safely help increase the metabolic rate and balance the glandular system.

Sassafras (*Sassafras officinale, Sassafras albidum, Sassafras variifolium, Laurus sassafras*)

Sassafras is a tree that has similar properties to cinnamon. It is alterative (balances bodily functions), aromatic, a stimulant and diaphoretic (promotes perspiration). It was used medicinally by native Americans for many centuries and it is said the aroma from the tree was what saved Columbus when he was trying to convince his mutinous crew that land was near. Unfortunately, one species that used to grow in North America is now extinct.

The root bark can be either chipped or crushed and then steeped in boiling water (one ounce of bark to one pint (0.47 litres) of water) and taken in doses of a wineglassful as often as needed.

Uses of sassafras

- Alleviates skin conditions
- Disinfectant in dental surgery
- Eases menstrual pain
- Prevents bladder stones
- Prevents and cures scurvy
- Prevents and treats oedema (inflammation)
- Reduces fevers
- Reduces labour pains

- Relieves eye inflammation
- Soothes rheumatism
- Treats gout.

Sassafras is often combined with guaiacum or sarsaparilla to treat bronchitis, chronic rheumatism, skin diseases and syphilis.

WARNING: Sassafras oil from the sassafras tree can produce narcotic poisoning and death by causing widespread fatty degeneration of the heart, liver, and kidneys, or, in a larger dose, by greatly reducing the circulation, followed by paralysing respiration. It should not be used by pregnant women as it can cause abortion.

Scutellaria (*Scutellaria baicalensis*, skullcap)

Scutellaria, also known as skullcap, is part of the *Lamiaceae* plant family and is a native of China. It is a very powerful antiviral herb with no side effects and is perfect for the treatment of pandemic diseases. The root of this plant, which has been used in Chinese medicine for a very long time as the herb Huang-qin, is extremely effective for treating contagious flu-like viruses. There is really no better anti-infection agent in the herb kingdom.

Scutellaria is also one of the most powerful herbs to induce sleep. It calms the nervous system, relaxes the muscles and helps balance blood pressure with no side effects. It also contains a compound known as baicalin that is as powerful as ibuprofen in reducing pain and inflammation, without the side effects.

The herb is more effective if grown in poor, sandy soil. Added advantages of scutellaria are:

- Quick to germinate
- Easily grown in most climates
- Can be harvested in the autumn of the first or second year.

Note: Avoid scutellaria if pregnant or breastfeeding.

Senega root (*Polygala vulgaris*, milkwort, rattlesnake root, seneca, snakeroot)

Senega root was highly esteemed by the native Seneca Indians for its effectiveness in curing rattlesnake bites and many other disorders. It is a diaphoretic (encourages sweating), cathartic (purifying), diuretic, expectorant and sialagogue (enhances saliva flow) and has emetic (stimulates vomiting) properties. It is especially effective for treating bronchitis and asthma by nourishing the respiratory tract. It is also useful for treating bleeding wounds, colds, emphysema, pain and inflammation, pneumonia and pleurisy, respiratory tract inflammation, rheumatism, tracheitis (inflammation of the trachea) and whooping cough.

It possesses an intricate blend of triterpenoid saponins in the roots that work by causing irritation locally on the stomach's internal coating and a nauseated feeling that eventually promotes secretions from the bronchial tubes as well as the sweat glands. However, care should be taken not to take this herb in excessive amounts, as it may result in violent purging and vomiting. It also contains phenolic acids, polygalitol, methyl salicylate and plant sterols.

It has been discovered that the saponins present in senega root hold promise as a treatment for type-2 diabetes.

The bark of *Polygala senega* is used to prepare a tea, which is drunk to induce abortions or cause miscarriage.

Note: Senega root can be poisonous when taken in large amounts and cause vomiting and aggressive purging. Excessive use may cause nervousness, vertigo and vision disturbance. People who are hypersensitive to salicylates or aspirin should stay away from using senega root. Pregnant women should also avoid this remedy.

Shiric sanango (*Brunfelsia grandiflora*)

In Pucallpa, Peru, a root infusion with aguardiente (an alcoholic beverage) of this Amazonian plant is taken to treat chills, rheumatism and venereal disease. The plant is regarded as diaphoretic (induces perspiration), diuretic, good to reduce fever and can be used to treat snakebites, syphilis and yellow fever. It contains lactic acid, quinic acid, scopoletin and tartaric acid.

Siberian ginseng (*Eleutherococcus senticosus*)

Siberian ginseng supports the glandular system. It is called an adaptogen, which means that it helps the body adapt to any situation which would normally alter its function. It has a beneficial effect on the heart and circulation and stimulates the entire body's energy production to overcome fatigue, stress and weakness. Studies suggest that it can also help reduce blood sugar levels, balance blood pressure and enhance the immune system by boosting the body's production of natural killer cells.

Note: Not recommended for patients with anxiety or high blood pressure.

Spring onions (*Allium cepa*, green onions, negi, naganegi)

Spring onions are immature onions and both the green and white parts of the vegetable are edible and should be used when being added to meals. Spring onions are a very good source of fibre, choline, vitamin A (retinol), vitamin B1 (thiamine), vitamin B2 (riboflavin), vitamin B3 (niacin), vitamin B9 (folate), vitamin C (ascorbic acid), vitamin E, vitamin K1, calcium, copper, iron, magnesium, manganese and potassium.

Note: As with onions, always leave spring onions for 10 minutes after chopping them to allow the production of the powerful antioxidant allicin to take place.

Stephania root (*Stephania tetrandra*, fang ji)

Stephania root has powerful antibacterial and anti-inflammatory properties. In Japan, it is used as a pain reliever and to treat inflammation and stiffness of the shoulders and back. In China, it is used to treat flatulence, kidney and spleen disorders and as an effective diuretic to relieve oedema. It is also known to be effective in treating Lyme disease and syphilis and can prevent silicosis. It can also help the cardiovascular system by increasing blood flow, expanding coronary vessels and lowering blood pressure.

Stone root (*Collinsonia canadensis*, Canada horsebalm, richweed, hardhack, heal-all, horseweed, ox balm)

This is a perennial medicinal herb in the mint family and its active components are mucilage, resins, saponins and tannins. It is useful for stabilising the lining of the sinuses and minimising the build-up of excess mucus in the nasal passages, stomach and throat. It also has the ability to relax painful constrictions and spasms of the rectum so it is used for anal fissures, fistulas and ulcers. It also has a relaxing effect on the urinary organs, where it can relax the ureter and therefore increase urination, reduce irritability of the bladder and assist with the passage of bladder and kidney stones.

Suma (*Pfaffia paniculata*, Brazilian ginseng)

In South America, suma is known as 'para todos' (which means: 'for all things') and as Brazilian ginseng, since it is widely used as an adaptogen with many applications (similar to ginseng). The indigenous peoples of the Amazon region have used suma root for generations for a wide variety of health purposes, including as a general tonic, an energy, rejuvenating and sexual tonic and as a general cure-all for many types of illness. Suma has been used as an aphrodisiac, a calming agent and to treat ulcers for at least 300 years. It is still an important herbal remedy of several Amazon rainforest indigenous tribes today.

Medicinal uses of suma

- Acts as an antibacterial and antifungal agent
- Balances blood sugar levels
- Enhances the immune system
- Enhances memory
- Helps to heal wounds
- Increases cellular oxygenation
- Increases oestrogen production
- Minimises the side effects of birth control medications
- Neutralises toxins
- Reduces high blood pressure and LDL cholesterol levels
- Reduces hormonal disorders and symptoms of menstruation and the menopause
- Restores glandular and nerve functions and balances the endocrine system
- Stimulates appetite and circulation
- Strengthens the muscular system
- Treats infertility.

Suma can also help to treat anaemia, anxiety and stress, arthritis, arteriosclerosis, bronchitis, cancer, circulatory and digestive disorders, diabetes, exhaustion, fatigue, impotence, inflammation, mononucleosis and rheumatism. It is also a helpful adjunct therapy in the treatment of syphilis and other sexually transmitted infections and as a general restorative tonic after illness.

As stated above, it is an adaptogen, which means it helps the body adapt to stress, and acts as a tonic to the entire system. By enhancing the body's immune system, suma helps prevent free-radical damage to the body. It contains significant amounts of germanium, a trace mineral which stimulates the immune system and helps promote oxygen flow to cells. It also contains allantoin, a substance which assists in healing wounds. Other beneficial nutrients include the natural plant hormones sitosterol and stigmasterol, which help to support circulatory and glandular systems.

The Japanese investigated suma in trials against specific types of tumour cells. The researchers discovered that six saponins called pffaffosides A, B, C, D, E, and F are the unique chemicals present that inhibit tumour cell growth. Brazilian researchers have found that suma is both safe and effective for altered-immune disorders.

Suma has also been called 'the Russian secret', as it has been taken by Russian Olympic athletes for many years and has been reported to increase muscle-building and endurance without the side effects associated with steroids. This action is attributed to an anabolic-type phytochemical called beta-ecdysterone and three novel ecdysteroid glycosides that are found in high amounts in suma.

A French company has also filed a US patent on the topical use of these ecdysterone chemicals, claiming that their suma ecdysterone extract strengthened the water barrier function of the skin, increased skin keratinocyte differentiation, which would be helpful for psoriasis, gave the skin a smoother, softer appearance and improved hair quality.

Suma root has a very high saponin content (up to 11%). One of the most famous plant saponins is digitalis, derived from the common foxglove, which has been used as a heart drug for over 100 years.

Note: The root powder has been reported to cause asthmatic allergic reactions if inhaled. Ingestion of large amounts of plant saponins in general (naturally occurring chemicals in suma) has shown to sometimes cause mild gastric disturbances, including nausea and stomach cramping. Reduce dosages if these side effects are noted. Avoid this plant if you are female and suffering from an oestrogen-positive cancer.

Swede (*Brassica napus*, rutabaga)

The word 'rutabaga' has been derived from the Swedish word 'rotabagge' where 'rota' means 'root'. Commonly known as swede, Swedish turnip or yellow turnip, rutabaga is a member of the Brassica family. Regular consumption of swede can increase milk production in lactating mothers. It can also increase and enhance stamina and digestion and helps to reduce wheezing in asthma patients, reduces the risk of cataract formation, supports the structure of capillaries, helps in decreasing stroke mortality, can lower high blood pressure and provides relief from constipation.

Swede also boosts the immune system, prevents cancer and heart disease and, when consumed by pregnant women before and during pregnancy, can prevent spina bifida in the newborn thanks to its folate content. It is also good to include in the diet when suffering from colds and coughs.

Swede can be baked, boiled and mashed, sautéed or steamed. It makes a great addition to soups and dishes with a little sweetness like honey or dried fruit. As a snack, cut the swede into cubes and steam until soft. Then toss the pieces with raisins, chopped walnuts and a little honey. It can also be served raw (if young and tender) in salads or chopped up and served with crunchy vegetables as a snack as it does not contain the poisonous solanine found in potatoes.

Swede is very low in calories and a good source of fibre and omega-3 and omega-6 fatty acids. It is high in carotene, vitamin C, vitamin B9 (folate), choline, calcium, magnesium, phosphorus and potassium. It also provides vitamin A (retinol), vitamin B1 (thiamine), vitamin B2 (riboflavin), vitamin B3 (niacin), vitamin B5 (pantothenic acid), vitamin E, vitamin K1, iron, sodium, zinc, copper, manganese and selenium.

Sweet potato (*Ipomoea batatas*)

The earliest cultivation records of the sweet potato date back to 750 BC in Peru, although archaeological evidence shows cultivation of the sweet potato may have begun around 2500-1850 BC. Sweet potatoes are related to morning glory and other vines. Although some people call them yams, true yams originated in China and are a different plant altogether, related to the lily.

Unlike white potatoes (see page 77), the leaves of which contain poisonous solanine, the leaves of the sweet potato plant are also edible and nutritious. Because white potatoes are members of the nightshade family, which some people have intolerances to, sweet potatoes are a good substitute. One study has shown that sweet potatoes reduce appetite and food intake which can be beneficial to individuals who are overweight.

Sweet potato provides 90 calories per 100 grams whereas white potatoes contain 70 calories. They also contain no saturated fats or cholesterol. In comparison with the white potato, they contain more fibre, iron, vitamins C, B9 and K and potassium but less sodium. They also contain betaine, choline and vitamins A, B1, B2, B3, B5, B6, D and E.

Sweet potatoes are extremely rich in minerals including: calcium, chromium, copper, germanium, iron, magnesium, manganese, molybdenum, nickel, phosphorus, potassium, selenium, silicon and zinc, which regulate and maintain the overall health of the body. Because they contain iron and help with the production of red and white blood cells, sweet potatoes can help to prevent and remedy anaemia. Their high dietary fibre content means they can prevent constipation and reduce the risk of colon cancer. Their high magnesium content helps the whole body and reduces stress. The magnesium and iron together help to reduce menstrual symptoms both before and during menstruation.

Sweet potatoes contain natural sugar, which controls and stabilises the sugar levels in the blood. Not only do they have a low glycaemic index, but they have been shown in a clinical trial to help reduce blood sugar levels and improve insulin sensitivity in adults with type-2 diabetes. This may be due to their chromium content.

The vitamin A in sweet potatoes can help to prevent retinal disorders that are common in people with diabetes. Vitamin A is also required by the body to maintain the integrity of healthy mucous membranes and skin. The anthocyanin in purple-skinned potatoes can reportedly reduce wrinkles, dark circles around eyes and puffy and swollen eyes. After boiling the potatoes with their skins on, keep the water and use it to clean the face for blemish-free healthy skin. Most smokers have a lack of vitamin A and have problems with emphysema (air sac damage). Sweet potatoes rejuvenate the respiratory system and prevent emphysema because of the high amounts of carotenoids that they contain. In total, 100 grams of the tuber provides 19,218 micrograms (µg) of vitamin A and 8509 µg of beta-carotene which also prevents hair damage and improves hair growth. The antioxidants beta-carotene, manganese, selenium and vitamins A, C and E, can improve the condition of the skin and help to treat arthritis, asthma and gout.

Sweet potatoes are extremely beneficial to consume during pregnancy because they also have high levels of folate, which is necessary for healthy foetal development.

They can help to control and maintain normal blood pressure and balance electrolytes due to their potassium content. Their high amount of vitamin B6 helps the function of the heart and to prevent heart attacks, strokes and digestive issues.

The vitamin D in sweet potatoes can help to support the immune system and is very important for maintaining the health of the thyroid gland, bones, teeth, skin and heart. Other components in sweet potatoes can also help to normalise the heart beat and the nerve signals that are sent to the brain. The germanium and selenium also help to build muscles and prevent muscle cramps and minimise inflammation and swelling.

A protein isolated from sweet potatoes has recently been shown to slow the growth of colon cancer cells by 65%. It also inhibited lung and oral cancers by 50%. Other lab research has shown that sweet potato also potently inhibits leukaemia, lymphoma and liver cancer cells. And in studies on humans, eating this vegetable, either alone or with other foods, has been associated with reducing the risk of kidney cancer by 56%, gallbladder cancer by 67% and breast cancer by 30%, when consumed three times a week. Sweet potatoes are rich in flavonoids which help to protect against all these cancers.

For the body to absorb the fat-soluble nutrients in sweet potatoes, such as carotenoids, they should always be consumed with an oily food such as avocado, butter or fish, nut, seed and other plant oils.

Sweet potatoes are rich in omega-6 fatty acids which are

inflammatory but low in omega-3 fatty acids which are anti-inflammatory, therefore the best way to consume them would be with a high omega-3 food to balance the ratio of these important fatty acids.

Highest sources of omega-3 fatty acids in milligrams per 100 grams to balance omega-6 fatty acids in sweet potato

- Krill oil 36,000 mg
- Flaxseed oil 22,813 mg
- Chia seeds 17,552 mg
- Walnuts 9079 mg
- Caviar (fish eggs) 6789 mg
- Cloves (ground) 4279 mg
- Oregano (dried) 4180 mg
- Marjoram (dried) 3230 mg
- Tarragon (dried) 2955 mg
- Mackerel 2670 mg
- Herring 2365 mg
- Salmon (wild) 2018 mg
- Lamb 1610 mg
- Basil (dried) 1509 mg
- Sardines 1480 mg
- Anchovies 1478 mg
- Soya beans 1433 mg
- Trout 1068 mg
- Pecans, sea bass 986 mg
- Pine nuts 787 mg
- Bell peppers (green) 770 mg
- Oysters 740 mg
- Radish seeds sprouted 722 mg
- Purslane 400 mg
- Basil (fresh leaves) 316 mg

- Rabbit 220 mg
- Kidney beans 194 mg
- Wakame seaweed 188 mg
- Alfalfa sprouts 175 mg
- Brussel sprouts 173 mg
- Rocket 170 mg
- Cauliflower 167 mg
- Spinach 138 mg
- Broccoli 129 mg
- Raspberries 126 mg
- Lettuce 113 mg
- Blueberries 94 mg
- Summer squash 82 mg
- Strawberries 65 mg
- Milk 75 mg
- Eggs 74 mg
- Chinese cabbage (pak choy) 55 mg
- Turnips 49 mg.

Tree turmeric (*Berberis aristata*, Indian berberry)

Tree turmeric is a Himalayan plant found between 2000 and 3000 metres above sea level. It contains calcium, iron, magnesium, pectin, phosphorus, potassium, vitamin C and tannins and, as the name suggests, tree turmeric has all of the qualities of normal turmeric. The root is one of the most successful medicines in India and its efficacy is almost equal to quinine but does not produce any adverse effects on the bowels, brain, stomach or affect the hearing as quinine can.

The dried extract of the roots is used to treat diseases related to the eyes, ears and face and is an excellent medication in the case of sun-blindness..

A tincture made from the root bark is used as a bitter tonic that has anti-periodic (prevents reoccurrences of infections), antipyretic (reduces fever), cholagogue (promotes the discharge of bile), purgative (blood purifying) and stomachic (promotes appetite and digestion) properties.

Medicinal uses of tree turmeric

- Colitis
- Diarrhoea
- Dysentery
- Eye infections
- Enlarged liver
- Gastroenteritis
- Heart failure
- Jaundice

- Malaria
- Menorrhagia (heavy menstrual bleeding)
- Periodic neuralgia
- Rheumatism
- Skin diseases
- Spleen disorders
- Trachoma.

The tree turmeric tincture can also be used topically for burns, glandular swellings, piles and sores and wounds to reduce inflammation and promote faster healing.

Tree turmeric also supports the immune system and is particularly good at reducing acquired intolerances or allergies. Acquired intolerances are allergic reactions to foods such as wheat or dairy that develop over time. These kinds of intolerance stem from an overactive immune system, with the root cause often being too many toxins in the body.

Turmeric (*Curcuma longa*)

Turmeric is the bright yellow of the spice rainbow. It is a powerful medicine that has long been used in the Chinese and Indian systems of medicine as an anti-inflammatory agent to treat a wide variety of conditions. Curcumin, the major constituent of turmeric that gives the spice its yellow colour, can correct the most common expression of the genetic defect that is responsible for cystic fibrosis. Curcumin exerts very powerful antioxidant effects that can neutralise free-radicals that can damage healthy cells and cell membranes. This is important in many diseases, such as arthritis, where free radicals are responsible for the painful joint inflammation and eventual damage to the joints.

Turmeric's combination of antioxidant and anti-inflammatory effects explains why many people with joint disease find relief when they use the spice regularly. Turmeric has also been scientifically proven to be more effective at treating depression than many common anti-depressant drugs.

Medicinal uses of turmeric

- Arthritis
- Bacterial infections
- Colic
- Depression
- Flatulence
- Hepatitis
- Jaundice and other liver disorders
- Menstrual disorders
- Neurological disorders
- Measles

- Toothache
- Ulcerative colitis
- Urinary infections
- Yeast infections

Turmeric can also provide an inexpensive, well-tolerated, and effective treatment for inflammatory bowel disease (IBD) such as Crohn's.

Treatment of brain cells, called astrocytes, with turmeric has been found to increase the expression of the amino acid glutathione and protect neurons exposed to oxidative stress. Glutathione can be beneficial for a huge range of diseases and disorders as it is present in every cell in the body and has an important antioxidant role.

The frequent consumption of turmeric has also been shown to lead to lower rates of breast, colon, lung and prostate cancers. Even when breast cancer is already present, curcumin can help slow the spread of breast cancer cells to the lungs. Prostate cancer is a rare occurrence among men in India, whose low risk is attributed to a diet rich in brassica family vegetables (cauliflower, cabbage, broccoli, Brussels sprouts, kale, kohlrabi and turnips) and the curry spice, turmeric. Both phenethyl isothiocyanate and curcumin greatly retard the growth of human prostate cancer cells. The combination of cruciferous vegetables and curcumin could be an effective therapy not only to prevent prostate cancer, but to inhibit the spread of established prostate cancers.

Recipe: Cauliflower spiced with turmeric

Cut cauliflower florets in quarters and let sit for 5-10 minutes; this allows time for the production of phenethyl isothiocyanates, which form when cruciferous vegetables are cut, but stops when they are heated. Then sprinkle with turmeric, and healthy sauté on medium heat in a few tablespoons of vegetable or chicken broth for five minutes. Remove from the heat and top with olive oil, sea salt and pepper to taste.

Recipe: Turmeric tea remedy

Turmeric makes an excellent antiseptic and anti-inflammatory tea. It can be used internally and externally to heal wounds, relieve pains in the limbs, break up congestion and as a restorative after the loss of blood from childbirth.

- In a pan place a quarter of 1 cup of water, ½ teaspoon turmeric, a pinch of black pepper and 3 cardamom pods (optional)
- Simmer for 5-7 minutes
- Then add 1 cup of milk and 2 tablespoons of almond or coconut oil (cold-pressed)
- Bring just to the boiling point (but do not boil)
- Add honey to taste
- Sip slowly as a hot tea.

Note: Avoid cumin, ginger and turmeric if taking:

- anticoagulants (blood thinning medication)
- hormone therapies
- contraceptive pills
- non-steroidal anti-inflammatory medications such as aspirin and ibuprofen, or
- have heart problems or
- during the first three months of pregnancy or
- are breast feeding.

Turnip (*Brassica rapa*)

Brassicas like turnips are a good source of carotenoids, fibre, indoles, omega-3 fatty acids, protein, vitamin A (retinol), vitamin B1 (thiamine), vitamin B2 (riboflavin), vitamin B3 (niacin), vitamin B5 (pantothenic acid), vitamin B6 (pyridoxine), vitamin B9, vitamin C (ascorbic acid), vitamin E, vitamin K and minerals such as calcium, copper, iron, magnesium, manganese, phosphorus, potassium and zinc.

Turnips, also known as 'neeps' in Scotland, can help to prevent blood clots and arterial blockages, reduce the risks of heart disease, fight bacterial, fungal and parasitic infections, prevent a variety of cancers, especially colorectal, and protect against the damage caused by nicotine.

Umbrella leaf (*Diphylleia cymosa*)

Umbrella root tea was used by the Cherokee tribe to induce

sweating. It has effects similar to the May apple (*Podophyllum peltatum*). Because of its rarity, little research has been carried out into its medicinal benefits. However, it is believed that the root might contain podophyllin, an effective anti-cancer agent.

Valerian root (*Valeriana officinalis*)

Valerian root can support the nervous system and has soothing properties. It is a safe and natural sleeping aid. Properties of the plant can give calming and relaxing relief to the blood vessels, muscles and nerves. Daily consumption of valerian will help to achieve a state of overall relaxation and elimination of stress which will, in turn, decrease blood pressure in people experiencing hypertension.

Violet tree root (*Securidaca longepedunculata*, krinkhout, mpesu, mamba)

The violet tree is a small tree, with fragrant purple flowers, indigenous to the tropical parts of Africa. The roots can treat a variety of physical and psychological problems such as discomfort, epilepsy, headaches, irritation and nervousness. It has been scientifically proven that the root extract is as powerful and effective as the pharmaceutical drug 'phenobarbitone' often used for epilepsy but without the damaging side effects.

Wafer ash (*Ptelea trifoliata*, hop tree, shrubby trefoil, stinking ash, swamp dogwood, wingseed)

The wafer ash is a shrub commonly found in hedges and woods in the United States. The decoction or tincture of the root bark is used to stimulate the appetite and for disorders of the digestive system as it can soothe the mucous membranes. It is said to have anthelmintic properties which means it can kill many parasites. It is used to treat asthma and other respiratory disorders, and intermittent fevers.

Note: Consumption of this remedy can cause inflammation of the skin but this will subside once treatment has stopped.

Wasabi (*Wasabia japonica*)

Wasabi is a paste made from the ground up root of this cruciferous Japanese vegetable. It has been used for centuries in Japan because it can kill harmful food-borne bacteria, reduce blood pressure, kill cancer cells, improve bone strength and liver function, detoxify the body of free radicals and improve gut function. It is naturally antiviral and antibacterial and stimulates the body's natural immune system.

Glucoraphanin, which transforms into sulforaphane in the body, is found in brassicas like wasabi and blocks a key destructive enzyme that damages cartilage. Consuming plenty of these cruciferous vegetables can protect the joints and help to treat arthritis. The sulphoraphane, in wasabi, also helps detoxification in the liver and may help to prevent breast cancer. Regular consumption of wasabi can boost the immune system, prevent spina bifida in newborns (if consumed during pregnancy) and prevent heart disease and many forms of cancer.

Wasabi may cause temporary inflammation of the throat and sinuses but can help to reduce inflammation in other parts of the body.

Note: Some unscrupulous restaurants and manufacturers will create a cheaper wasabi substitute from mustard, horseradish and food colourings. This does not provide the same set of nutritional benefits as real wasabi so care needs to be taken to ensure that the wasabi being consumed is actually from the wasabi plant itself.

Wild yam (*Dioscorea oppositae*)

Wild yam has many effective uses. It is known to relax the muscles and promote glandular balance in women. It contains natural plant components ('phytonutrients') which help the body balance hormone levels so is especially useful during the menopause by helping to eliminate hot flushes. It also supports the digestive system and the nerves and is helpful to the liver and endocrine system.

Yacon root (*Smallanthus sonchifolius*, Peruvian ground apple)

Yacon is a perennial plant in the *Asteraceae* family that is mainly cultivated for its sweet-flavoured roots. It is mainly grown in the northern and central Andes but has also been introduced into countries like Australia and New Zealand where the climate is mild and the growing season long. Today, it is also grown in home gardens in some parts of the US and UK and may be found in some farmers' markets. Raw yacon has a crunchy texture and is good peeled, diced and eaten as a snack or added to salads. As with most light-coloured root vegetables, it should be peeled, sliced and placed in water that contains lemon juice or apple cider vinegar to prevent discolouration.

Yacon root is a rich source of the prebiotic substance inulin, which supports bone health, immune function and gut bacteria balance by encouraging a healthy intestinal environment. It also promotes normal development of epithelial tissue, supports absorption of calcium and magnesium, stabilises blood sugar levels, supports immune cell function and antibody production in the gut, promotes a healthy pH in the lower gastrointestinal tract, promotes healthy elimination of waste and is an excellent source of fibre.

Yams (*Dioscorea alata*)

Yams, often confused with sweet potatoes, are a tuber native to Africa and Asia and are closely related to lilies. They vary in size from equivalent to a small potato to a record 130 pounds (as of 1999) and are generally cylindrical in shape. Yam flesh ranges in colour from tan to pink or purple and tends to be dry and starchy.

Yams contain just 35 calories per 100 grams, making them a good choice for individuals wanting to lose weight. They can be eaten raw in salads and replacing potatoes with yams can provide more fibre and antioxidants to the diet. They are an excellent source of antioxidants, minerals and vitamins.

Fresh yam tubers are prebiotic being an excellent source of oligofructose and inulin, which belong to a class of carbohydrates known as fructans and soluble dietary fibre that feed the beneficial bacteria in the colon. Inulin is a zero-calorie, sweet-tasting, inert carbohydrate that does not metabolise in the human body, which makes the root an ideal sweet snack for diabetics and dieters plus its components offer protection from cancers, inflammation and viral coughs and colds. They also help to keep the cells of the colon healthy, preventing such conditions as colon cancer, diverticular disease and ulcerative colitis. They also help regulate cholesterol and insulin levels, protect from heart disease and relieve premenstrual tension.

Yams are rich in vitamin C, copper, iron, magnesium and manganese. They also contain small levels of vitamin B1 (thiamine), vitamin B2 (riboflavin), vitamin B5 (pantothenic acid), vitamin B6 (pyridoxine) and vitamin B9 (folate).

Yellow dock root (*Rumex crispus*)

Yellow dock is a bitter herb noted for its high iron content. It is therefore good for treating anaemia. It nourishes the skin, stimulates bile production, helps the function of the gallbladder and purifies the blood. It is also known to treat impotence and bacterial orchitis.

Zhi mu (*Anemarrhena asphodeloides*)

The zhu mui root, also known as 'common *Anemarrhena*', rhizome is used in traditional Chinese medicine and usually cooked in boiling water to make tea or soup for consumption daily of between 6 and 12 milligrams depending on the health issue and person consuming it.

Internally, zhi mu is used for high fever in chronic bronchitis, infectious diseases, tuberculosis and urinary problems. In Chinese herbal medicine, it is used for coughs, fever and night sweats, particularly in combination with rehmannia and the Chinese figwort (*Scrophularia ningpoensis*). Externally, it is used to treat mouth ulcers.

It has an antibacterial action, inhibiting the growth of *Bacillus dysenteriae*, *B. typhi*, *B. paraatyphi*, *Proteus* and *Pseudomonas*. Externally, it is used as a mouthwash in the treatment of ulcers. The rhizome is harvested in the autumn and dried for later use. Therapeutic action is slightly altered by cooking with wine or salt. **Note:** Zhi mu should not be given to patients with diarrhoea and should be administered with caution since, when taken in excess (more than 6-12 milligrams per day), it can cause a sudden drop in blood pressure.

Prebiotic roots

Many roots are a prebiotic food containing carbohydrates, such as inulin, that encourages a healthy intestinal environment to benefit probiotic intestinal gut bacteria. 'Prebiotic' is a fairly recently coined name to refer to food components that support the growth of certain kinds of bacteria (probiotics) in the colon (large intestine). Oligosaccharides, resistant starch and fermentable fibre feed these probiotic bacteria which have an important influence on the rest of the body; all these substances can be found in certain root vegetables.

The human digestive system has a hard time breaking down many of these carbohydrates. Almost 90 per cent escape digestion in the small intestine and reach the colon intact; this is where they become prebiotic. The bacteria that reside in the colon feed on fermentable carbohydrates and produce many beneficial substances, including short-chain fatty acids, vitamin A, vitamin K2 and certain B vitamins. They also promote further absorption of some minerals that have escaped the small intestine, including calcium and magnesium. Vitamin K2 is produced by these bacteria using vitamin K1 in the diet and is essential for the human body to direct calcium to the bones. Without it calcium remains in the blood and can cause problems such as calcium oxalate stones in the bladder, gall bladder and kidneys and calcified plaques in blood vessels. At the same time, bones can become brittle and porous due to the lack of calcium, leading to osteoporosis.

Ingredients

- Unrefined sea salt/Himalayan pink salt (not iodised salt)
- Filtered or bottle mineral water
- Herbs and spices such as anise seeds, bay leaves, cardamom seeds, cumin, dill, garlic, ginger, marjoram, nasturtium, nutmeg, tarragon, turmeric or vanilla. (Use according to taste but use no more than three dominant, complementary flavours. Experiment and create pickles based on nutritionally beneficial or medicinal vegetables, herbs and spices (see *Nature Cures – the A-Z of Ailments and Natural Foods*) for a particular condition or for taste. For example, beetroot is good with hard boiled eggs, onion, cloves and dill.)

Method

1. Mix salt and water to make a 5%-salt solution (brine). If you need 2 litres of water to cover the vegetables, you will use 100 grams of salt, for example. You need enough water to completely cover all the vegetables, so how much water and salt you need depends on the volume of vegetables being used.
2. In a sterilised pickling jar, layer the well-washed and prepared vegetables and spices.
3. Leave about 5 cm (2 inches) at the top.
4. Whisk the brine well to completely dissolve the salt and pour it over the vegetables to just cover them.

5. Weigh down the vegetables to keep them fully submerged in the brine by using a plate that just fits inside the container, creating a seal, and weight the plate down with a well-scrubbed, large rock or a slightly smaller container that has been filled with water.

6. Alternately, use a plastic bag filled with brine to act as both a weight and a seal. Do this by fitting a heavy plastic freezer bag inside another. Fill the inner bag with a salt brine of three tablespoons salt to one litre of water and tightly close both bags to prevent leaks. Place on top of the pickles, making sure it fits tightly around the inner edge of the jar. It acts as an airtight weight on top of the vegetables, which will discourage the growth of yeast and scum.

7. Store the pickles in a cool (15-23°C (60-75°F)) place. Liquid may bubble and seep from the pickles as they ferment, so place the pickle container on a tray or in a bowl to contain any overflow.

8. The pickles will take about four to 10 days to complete fermentation, depending on the temperature of fermentation and the concentration of salt in the brine. Cooler temperatures and saltier brines slow fermentation. The fermentation is complete when bubbles are no longer rising to the surface of the pickles and they have a fresh, tart smell. Taste the brine. If the saltiness is not balanced with sourness, let the pickles continue to ferment another day or two.

9. The pickles will keep for up to a year in the refrigerator as long as they remain submerged in the brine.

Index

Note: Some beneficial plant properties, such as anti-inflammatory, antibacterial and antiviral actions and help with fever, coughs and rheumatism, are shared by so many of the roots in this book that there would be no value in including them in the index. Therefore only specific conditions have been listed.

About the Author

Nat H Hawes SNHS Dip. (Advanced Nutrition and Sports Nutrition) has been studying and researching natural remedies, nutrients and the power of traditional foods and medicines since 2003. She believes, based on this research, that, unless nutrient deficiencies are tested for properly and shown to be present, extracted nutrient supplements are unnecessary and can do more harm than good. Natural and unrefined whole foods will provide the body with all the fuel it requires to function correctly and recover from most common ailments. She can be contacted through the following:

- Website: naturecures.co.uk
- Email: health@naturecures.co.uk
- Mobile: +44 (0)7966 519844